Preimplantation Genetic Testing

Preimplantation Genetic Testing
Recent Advances in Reproductive Medicine

Edited by

Darren K. Griffin, BSc, PhD, PGCertHE, CBiol, FRSA, FRSB, FRCPath, DSc

Professor of Genetics, School of Biosciences
Director, Centre for Interdisciplinary Studies of Reproduction
University of Kent
Canterbury, United Kingdom

Gary L. Harton, PhD

Global Director, Market Development PGT
PerkinElmer, Inc.
Waltham, Massachusetts, USA
Honorary Senior Lecturer, University of Kent
Canterbury, United Kingdom
Teacher, Eastern Virginia Medical School
Norfolk, Virginia, USA
Teacher, Bryant University
Smithfield, Rhode Island, USA

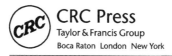

CRC Press
Taylor & Francis Group
Boca Raton London New York

CRC Press is an imprint of the
Taylor & Francis Group, an **informa** business

First edition published 2020
by CRC Press
6000 Broken Sound Parkway NW, Suite 300, Boca Raton, FL 33487-2742

and by CRC Press
2 Park Square, Milton Park, Abingdon, Oxon, OX14 4RN

© 2020 by Taylor & Francis Group, LLC

CRC Press is an imprint of Taylor & Francis Group, LLC

ISBN: 978-1-138-33341-3 (hbk)
ISBN: 978-1-138-33330-7 (pbk)
ISBN: 978-0-429-44597-2 (ebk)

Typeset in Times LT Std
by Nova Techset Private Limited, Bengaluru and Chennai, India.

Visit the Taylor & Francis Web site at
http://www.taylorandfrancis.com

and the CRC Press Web site at
http://www.crcpress.com

Contents

Foreword

Thirty years on from the first pregnancies and live births following IVF, embryo biopsy, and single-cell genetic analysis in couples at risk of X-linked diseases [1], preimplantation genetic diagnosis (PGD), or preimplantation genetic testing for monogenic disease (PGT-M), as it has recently been renamed, is now well established as a valuable alternative to prenatal diagnosis for a wide range of inherited conditions [2,3].

In the early days, embryos could only be cultured for 2 or 3 days post insemination (Day 2 or 3) before they were transferred to the uterus, and even delaying transfer to Day 4 reduced implantation and pregnancy rates. The slow freezing protocols used for cryopreservation of embryos at these early stages were rudimentary, and often embryos were destroyed or partially damaged in the thawing process. The challenge, therefore, was to remove a single cell from each embryo early on Day 3 at the 6- to 10-cell stage to minimize the damage to the embryo, perform the genetic analysis for the mutation on single copies of the parents' chromosomes within a few hours, and then select unaffected embryos for transfer later the same day. This could only be contemplated because of the emergence in the mid-1980s of the polymerase chain reaction (PCR), which allowed the million-fold amplification of short fragments of DNA. In addition, human genetics was still in its infancy and the mutations causing only a handful of common inherited diseases had been identified.

Today, there have been major advances in all aspects of preimplantation genetics that have revolutionized our ability to interrogate the genetics of human gametes and embryos. Embryo culture to the blastocyst stage on Days 5 to 7 and biopsy of multiple trophectoderm cells using laser-assisted hatching and excision is now routine. Cryopreservation of biopsied blastocysts, using ultra-rapid freezing, or vitrification, is highly efficient and minimally damaging, removing any time constraints on the genetic analysis. Most importantly, the ability to amplify the whole genome of single or small numbers of cells efficiently and generate micrograms of DNA has revolutionized our ability to perform genetic tests enabling the use of genome-wide methods including microarrays and next-generation sequencing (NGS). Alongside these developments, the sequencing of the human genome in the early 2000s and progress in identifying the genetic basis of thousands of monogenic diseases and other conditions has expanded the range of applications for PGT. These include rare severe childhood lethal diseases, late-onset diseases, genetic predisposition to cancers, and tissue typing to enable cord blood stem cells to be used for transplantation to existing affected children in the family.

Chromosome aneuploidy is a major cause of pregnancy failure and loss following natural conception. The use of various molecular cytogenetic methods for PGT of aneuploidy (PGT-A) has confirmed the high incidence of aneuploidy in human gametes and embryos, particularly in oocytes in which the incidence increases exponentially in women above the age of 35 years. PGT-A following blastocyst biopsy is therefore widely used for euploid embryo selection for infertile patients and there is accumulating evidence for significantly improved implantation rates and live birth outcomes, particularly following single vitrified-warmed embryo transfer in later managed cycles. However, the use of quantitative, mainly NGS-based methods, for 24-chromosome copy number analysis has revealed a relatively high incidence of intermediate copy number changes interpreted as indicating mosaicism for aneuploidies among the sampled trophectoderm cells. The clinical significance of low-level mosaicism is not fully understood since there are now reports of apparently healthy live births following transfer of embryos with only this type of copy number change. One explanation is that the affected trophectoderm cells may not be representative of the inner cell mass from which the fetus is derived. Alternatively, these cells may simply not be viable, and die out during early development.

Inherited diseases typically affect all the cells and tissues of the body, and the clinical manifestations are often multisystemic. This makes them challenging to treat. However, there has been some progress. For example, there is now a drug that can effectively arrest the neurological degeneration in children affected by Batten disease [4] and there has been some success with gene therapy for beta thalassemia [5]. However, these therapies remain highly expensive and limited in their availability. For couples who know that they are at risk of having affected children either because of a clinical diagnosis in an existing child or family member or increasingly because of the availability of preconception screening for extensive panels of serious recessive monogenic diseases, PGT or prenatal diagnosis following natural conception remain the only options for them to have their own healthy children.

Thirty years ago, it was anticipated that early noninvasive methods of diagnosing inherited disease from trophoblast cells recovered from the lower pole of the uterus or from cell-free fetal DNA in maternal blood would be developed and would, within a few years, replace PGT because of the expense and difficulty of the IVF process, especially for fertile couples. In the event, it would be over two decades later following the development of NGS that noninvasive prenatal testing (NIPT) for common aneuploidies became possible and only now that this approach is being extended to genome-wide aneuploidies, microdeletion syndromes, and some monogenic diseases [6].

Live birth rates following IVF have increased steadily over the last 30 years with improvements to culture media and laboratory conditions, and with PGT-A, implantation rates per embryo transfer can now average 60%–80% irrespective of maternal age. In the early years, many women in their 40s having PGT-M had repeated cycles without success, presumably because the majority or all of the unaffected embryos that were transferred had one or more aneuploidies and were not viable. Today, using combined PGT-M and aneuploidy testing (PGT-M/A), clinical outcomes are similarly improved by transferring only euploid-unaffected embryos, and patients can make an informed choice about continuing treatment.

Preimplantation genetic testing remains technically challenging and demanding and requires a multidisciplinary team, including expert genetic counseling to ensure the couple are fully aware of their options and the possible outcomes. Nevertheless, the birth of thousands of unaffected children worldwide is a testament to the value couples place on starting a pregnancy knowing that it is unaffected, and a reward for all the dedicated work of those involved in helping them to have healthy children.

Alan H. Handyside
School of Biosciences
University of Kent
Canterbury, United Kingdom

REFERENCES

1. Handyside AH, Kontogianni EH, Hardy K, Winston RML. Pregnancies from biopsied human preimplantation embryos sexed by Y-specific DNA amplification. *Nature*. 1990;344.
2. Handyside AH. 'Designer babies' almost thirty years on. *Reproduction*. 2018;156:F75–9.
3. Niederberger C et al. Forty years of IVF. *Fertil Steril*. 2018;110:185–324.e5.
4. Kohlschütter A, Schulz A, Bartsch U, Storch S. Current and emerging treatment strategies for neuronal ceroid lipofuscinoses. *CNS Drugs*. 2019;33:315–25.
5. Ikawa Y, Miccio A, Magrin E, Kwiatkowski JL, Rivella S, Cavazzana M. Gene therapy of hemoglobinopathies: Progress and future challenges. *Hum Mol Gen*. 2019;28(R1):R24–30.
6. Hayward J, Chitty LS. Beyond screening for chromosomal abnormalities: Advances in non-invasive diagnosis of single gene disorders and fetal exome sequencing. *Semin Fetal Neonatal Med*. 2018;23:94–101.

Editors

Darren K. Griffin earned his Bachelor of Science and Doctor of Science degrees from the University of Manchester and his PhD from University College London. After postdoctoral stints at Case Western Reserve University (Cleveland, Ohio) and the University of Cambridge, he had his first academic post at Brunel University (London), before settling at the University of Kent (Canterbury, United Kingdom), where he has worked for over 15 years. He has worked under the mentorship of Professors Joy Delhanty, Christine Harrison, Terry Hassold, Alan Handyside, and Malcolm Ferguson-Smith.

He is president of the International Chromosome and Genome Society and a Fellow of the Royal College of Pathologists, the Royal Society of Biology, and the Royal Society for the Encouragement of Arts, Manufactures and Commerce. He sits on the faculty of CoGEN (Controversies in Genetics) and has previously sat on the board of the Preimplantation Genetic Diagnosis International Society (PGDIS), organizing its annual meeting in 2014.

Professor Griffin is a world leader in cytogenetics. He performed the first successful cytogenetic PGD (using X and Y FISH probes for sexing) and, more recently, played a significant role in the development of karyomapping, an approach he now applies to cattle. Throughout a scientific research career of over 30 years he has co-authored over 200 scientific publications, mainly on the cytogenetics of reproduction and evolution, most recently providing insight into the karyotypes of dinosaurs.

He is a prolific science communicator, making every effort to make scientific research publicly accessible (both his own and others') and is an enthusiastic proponent for the benefits of interdisciplinary research endeavours. He has supervised over 35 PhD students to completion, and his work appears consistently in the national and international news. He currently runs a vibrant research lab of about 20 people (including a program of externally supervised students) and maintains commercial interests in the outcomes of research findings, liaising with companies in the field.

Gary L. Harton earned his Bachelor of Science degree from James Madison University (Harrisonburg, Virginia) and his PhD at the University of Kent (Canterbury, United Kingdom). His thesis title was "Facilitating the widespread use of preimplantation genetic diagnosis and screening through best practice and novel technology development."

After more than 20 years serving in various roles, including both clinical laboratory and management positions, he began his commercial career performing business development and market development roles with two prominent genetics companies, a fertility startup and a large reference genetics laboratory. Dr. Harton has been involved in a number of exciting breakthroughs in the field of reproductive genetics, including performing the first clinical preimplantation genetic diagnosis (PGD) for an autosomal dominant disease (Marfan syndrome) and performing the first clinical PGD for spinal muscular atrophy (SMA). In addition, Dr. Harton was involved in the team that pioneered non-disclosing Huntington disease (HD) PGD, where a patient at risk for HD could ensure that their children were free from the mutation without discovering their own HD status. He was also involved in the team that discovered and patented karyomapping, a revolutionary new technology allowing practically any genetic defect to be diagnosed in embryos using one single array-based test.

Dr. Harton is certified by the American Board of Bioanalysis (ABB) as a technical supervisor in molecular diagnostics and is a member of the American Society for Reproductive Medicine (ASRM) as well as the European Society of Human Reproduction and Embryology (ESHRE), and the Preimplantation Genetic Diagnosis International Society (PGDIS). Dr. Harton is currently a member of the board of directors for PGDIS and a member of the Special Advisory Group for United Kingdom-NEQAS, which performs external quality assessment schemes for preimplantation genetics. He has also served as chair of the Steering Committee for the ESHRE PGD and has been an author on numerous peer-reviewed scientific articles, abstracts, and book chapters.

Contributors

Lauri D. Black
Pacific Reproductive Genetic Counseling
Pacifica, California

Alison Campbell
CARE Fertility
Nottingham, United Kingdom

Antonio Capalbo
Igenomix
Marostica (VI), Italy

and

Dipartimento di Scienze Anatomiche, Istologiche
Medico-Legali e dell'Apparato Locomotore
Sezione Istologia ed Embriologia Medica
Sapienza University of Rome
Rome, Italy

Martine De Rycke
Centre for Medical Genetics
Universitair Ziekenhuis Brussel
and
Reproduction and Genetics
Vrije Universiteit Brussel (VUB)
Brussels, Belgium

Francesco Fiorentino
GENOMA Group
Molecular Genetics Laboratories
Rome and Milan, Italy

Jill M. Fischer
New Jersey Center for Science, Technology &
    Mathematics (NJCSTM)
Kean University
Union, New Jersey

Carmen María García-Pascual
R&D Department
Igenomix & Igenomix Foundation
INCLIVA
Valencia, Spain

Ermanno Greco
Reproductive Medicine
European Hospital
Rome, Italy

Darren K. Griffin
Centre for Interdisciplinary Studies of
Reproduction (CISoR)
School of Biosciences
University of Kent
Canterbury, United Kingdom

Alan H. Handyside
Centre for Interdisciplinary Studies of
Reproduction (CISoR)
School of Biosciences
University of Kent
Canterbury, United Kingdom

Anver Kuliev
Department of Human and Medical
    Genetics
Herbert Wertheim College of Medicine
Florida International University
Miami, Florida
and
Reproductive Genetic Innovations (RGI)
Northbrook, Illinois

Lucía Martínez-Merino
R&D Department
Igenomix
Valencia, Spain

Maria Giulia Minasi
Reproductive Medicine
European Hospital
Rome, Italy

Luis Navarro-Sánchez
R&D Department
Igenomix
Valencia, Spain

Cagri Ogur
Bahçeci Genetic Diagnosis Center
Altunizade
and
Department of Bioengineering
Yildiz Technical University
İstanbul, Turkey

Maurizio Poli
Igenomix
Marostica (VI), Italy

and

REPROOMICS
Amsterdam, Netherlands

Svetlana Rechitsky
Department of Human and Medical
    Genetics
Herbert Wertheim College of Medicine
Florida International University
Miami, Florida

and

Reproductive Genetic Innovations (RGI)
Northbrook, Illinois

Carmen Rubio
R&D Department
Igenomix & Igenomix Foundation
INCLIVA
Valencia, Spain

Carlos Simón
R&D Department
Igenomix
and
Department of Obstetrics and Gynaecology
Valencia University
and
Igenomix Foundation
INCLIVA
Valencia, Spain

and

Department of Obstetrics and Gynecology
School of Medicine
Stanford University
Stanford, California

Joe Leigh Simpson
Department of Human and Medical Genetics
Herbert Wertheim College of Medicine
Florida International University
Miami, Florida

and

Reproductive Genetic Innovations (RGI)
Northbrook, Illinois

Francesca Spinella
GENOMA Group
Molecular Genetics Laboratories
Rome and Milan, Italy

Alan Thornhill
Centre for Interdisciplinary Studies of
    Reproduction
School of Biosciences
University of Kent
Canterbury, United Kingdom

and

Igenomix United Kingdom, Ltd
Surrey, United Kingdom

Olga Tsuiko
Laboratory of Cytogenetics and Genome Research
Department of Human Genetics
KU Leuven
Leuven, Belgium

Pieter Verdyck
Centre for Medical Genetics
Universitair Ziekenhuis Brussel
Reproduction and Genetics
and
Vrije Universiteit Brussel (VUB)
Brussels, Belgium

Joris Robert Vermeesch
Laboratory of Cytogenetics and Genome Research
Department of Human Genetics
KU Leuven
Leuven, Belgium

Kateřina Veselá
REPROMEDA Biology Park
Brno, Czech Republic

Andrea Victor
Centre for Interdisciplinary Studies of
    Reproduction
School of Biosciences
University of Kent
Canterbury, United Kingdom

and

Zouves Fertility Center
Foster City, California

1

Preimplantation Genetic Testing and Reproductive Genetics from a Physician's Perspective

Kateřina Veselá

CONTENTS

Introduction

Reproductive genetics is now inseparably linked to reproductive medicine procedures and is becoming an integral part thereof. It has been applied in the diagnosis of factors of infertility and genetic disorder carrier status. This is specifically used for screening assessments before admitting a couple to an *in vitro* fertilization (IVF) program for targeted diagnosis of hereditary diseases or defects, or as part of preimplantation genetic testing (PGT) procedures. In many cases it is becoming an integral part of controlling therapeutic results in the form of noninvasive or invasive prenatal diagnosis.

Reproductive-genetic counseling in infertile couples is a comprehensive communication process purposed to evaluate a risk for genetic disorder in an offspring and to discuss measures to minimize that risk and improve the results of the treatment. Options for optimal testing and screening, interpretation and implications of test results, further education about a potential genetic diagnosis and prognosis, and emotional support are highly important aspects of a reproductive-genetic counseling visit. The core ethical principles of genetic counseling are the autonomy of the individual or couple, their right to full information, and the highest standards of confidentiality.

Although crude monetary arguments are not generally used to justify the provision of genetic counseling services, financial analysis might show a net cost savings to society/family by the reduction of expenditure on caring for those with serious genetic disease or disability.

Our contemporary professional goals in reproductive genetics are quite different from former ideas of eugenic medicine ("the health of the people," i.e., of the race). Respect for individual autonomy takes precedence over measures of the impact of genetic services on the population. We have always to comply with the wish for having a healthy baby, which is universal in all couples. Reproductive genetics is a part of medicine whose general purpose is to prevent or at least minimize suffering and distress.

Cytogenetic Testing

Basic cytogenetic tests used in reproductive medicine include karyotyping, performed for many years using G-banding [1] in cultured peripheral blood cells (lymphocytes). One of the best-established means of genetic diagnosis, adaptations of the original approach are used to this day, supplemented by enhanced banding techniques and digitized analysis. Given the dynamic development of molecular biology, this method has, in part, been successfully converted to a molecular genetic platform for routine use in a short time horizon. Currently, flatbed microarrays and the single nucleotide polymorphism (SNP) array method [2] are used for closer specifications of the findings of classical karyotyping if there are any unclear aspects, and in special indications. Microarrays provide considerably higher resolving power compared to G-banding, and can be used to detect microdeletions or microduplications as low as 0.5 Mb.

Expanded carrier screening (ECS) of patients as well as gamete donation is performed ever more commonly as part of testing before inclusion in the IVF program. Similarly, as in the case of new preimplantation and prenatal testing methods, the development of ECS has been made possible by the arrival of newer developments in molecular genetics [3].

Multiple-Gene NGS Panels

The introduction of next-generation sequencing (NGS) (including massive parallel sequencing [MPS]) has allowed a substantially wider and more detailed analysis of the genetic causes and relationships of pathological conditions [4]. Multiple-gene panels allow testing of many genes in a very short time. Such panels are typically a set of genes tested in parallel; physically, it is a set of DNA segments used to prepare a library, subsequently used as the basis for sequencing [5,6].

Tests using multiple-gene panels are most commonly used in oncology to detect inherited mutations in oncogenes [7], and in cardiological diagnosis [8]. Currently, their use is rapidly increasing for use in reproductive medicine [4–6]. Some reproductive clinics use standardized commercial panels, while others design an individual structure and assign the production of panels created based on their own specific requirements.

The purpose of using panels in modern reproductive medicine is to determine any potential genetic causes of fertility disorders in the man and woman, to uncover any gene mutations that might lead to the development of serious inherited diseases in the offspring, and finally to detect any factors posing potential risks to infertility therapy which could have potentially adverse impacts on the result.

Regularly tested gene mutations that cause the most common serious inherited diseases include mutations in the CFTR gene causing cystic fibrosis, the SMN1 gene causing spinal muscular atrophy, the GJB2 gene causing nonsyndromic deafness, and the FMR1 gene causing fragile X syndrome. Sites in different countries may include isolated tests of various mutations or implement these in multiple-gene panels with respect to habitual practice, patient requirements, legal regulations, or guidelines of a local professional association.

Description of Molecular Genetic Methods Used in the "PANDA" Panel Clinically at Repromeda, Brno, Czech Republic

The scientists and clinicians at Repromeda have developed a custom NGS panel that assesses a number of specific mutations as noted previously. Details of this test, called PANDA, are included next to highlight one specific use of custom panels used during an IVF cycle.

In brief, the test includes steps for performing preparation of the library: Custom Amplicon Library NEXTFlex NOVA-4301-03 Bioo Scientific Corp. (Perkin Elmer), sequencing using the MiSeq system (Illumina), evaluation using SeqPilot software (JSI Medical Systems), Repromeda bioinformatics software—SOP00417.

Additional detection test (CGG)n—Fragile X, Repromeda CGG RP PCR detection and AmplideX FMR1 PCR Kit® (Asuragen), fragmentation analysis—SOP 00415. This is a diagnostic genetic test designed for the testing of mutations that cause the most common genetic diseases in the Central European population; furthermore, thrombophilic mutations and genes/variants clinically related to infertility, hormonal stimulation, embryonal development, and pregnancy losses are tested.

Cystic Fibrosis

The 5'UTR region of the CFTR gene, the entire coding region of the gene CFTR±10 bp exon/intron overlap, poly-T/TG allelic variant in intron 8, mutations of CFTRdele2,3 kb, 1811+1,6 kbA>G, 3272−26A>G and 3849+10 kbC>T mutation are tested. The testing cannot detect changes in copy number variants (CNV) of individual exons except the deletion of exons 2 and 3 (mutation CFTRdele2,3,kb), or intra-gene rearrangements in the CFTR gene. If the test result is negative (i.e., no evidence of carrier status), the residual risk for the presence of a pathogenic variant in the CFTR gene in the subject is ≈ 1:900.

Besides its application for excluding the risk of cystic fibrosis being passed to the next generation, CFTR gene testing is also important in the diagnosis of male infertility. Mutations can cause congenital absence of the vas deferens (bi- or unilateral), bilateral obstruction of the ductus ejaculatorius, or bilateral obstruction of the ductus epididymis. All men with idiopathic obstructive azoospermia should thus have their CFTR gene examined.

Spinal Muscular Atrophy

Deletion of exons 7 and 8 of the SMN1 gene is tested, as this deletion is present in most carriers of spinal muscular atrophy. The testing is associated with 5% false negative results. Carriers exist who have two copies of exons 7 and 8 of the SMN1 gene on one chromosome and no copy on the other chromosome, which cannot be differentiated using any available method. Approximately 6% of patients with SMA may have a *de novo* deletion or another congenital intra-gene mutation in the SMN1 gene. If the test result is negative (no evidence of carrier status), the residual risk for the presence of a pathogenic variant in the SMN1 gene in the subject is ≈ 1:1500.

Deafness (Mutation in Connexin 26)

We test the entire coding region of the GJB2 gene, which has only one exon. The test cannot detect changes in the CNVs of the GJB2 gene and/or any intra-gene rearrangements. If the test result is negative (no evidence of carrier status), the residual risk for the presence of a pathogenic variant in the GJB2 gene in the subject is ≈ 1:740.

Fragile X Syndrome

We test CGG repeats in the FMR1 gene. According to the European Society of Human Genetics, (CGG) n < 45 is a normal finding, the range of 45–54 is a normal finding in the "grey zone," 55–200 means premutation, and n > 200 is full mutation. FMR1 gene mutation testing falls both in the group of gene mutation tests and of infertility cause tests given that premature ovarian failure is more common in female carriers of the premutation, and therefore decreased ovarian reserve in young women should also be an indication for the testing of this gene.

Additional genes tested in the previously named panel include thrombophilic mutations—coagulation factor V Leiden mutation (G169A) and R2 (H1299R) mutation; factor II prothrombin (G2021A mutation); MTHFR (methylene tetrahydrofolate reductase—C667T and A1298C mutations); plasminogen activator inhibitor PAI-I (haplotype 4G/5G); annexin 5 (ANXA5—M2 haplotype). Furthermore, we test the HSPA4L variant (PLK4 variant) where certain genotypes are associated with an increased risk of embryonic mosaicism.

Although there is no clear evidence of MTHFR gene variants having an impact on thrombophilia and in this respect can be understood as an adjuvant factor, the C677T variant is associated with an increased risk of embryo aneuploidy [9]. Thus, in this respect, it is not merely a negligible variant of the norm as declared in recent years, but instead a potentially significant indicator of reproductive risk, and further studies are needed for clarification.

Furthermore, the panel includes prediction of response to hormonal stimulation where individual variants are tested that are associated with various degrees of sensitivity of the follicle-stimulating hormone (FSH) receptor (Ser680Asn and c.-29G>A), luteinizing chorionic gonadotropic hormone (insLQp.18 and Asn291Ser), and the luteinizing hormone subunit beta (LHB) v-LHβ (c.82T>C & c.104T>C).

Mutations in the androgenic receptor and microdeletions in chromosome Y (AZFa, AZFb, AZFc) are tested in infertile men.

Diagnosis of Other Potential Fertility Disorders

A considerable number of fertility disorders are genetically determined [10]; moreover, some fertility disorders are related to the development of genetic defects in the offspring.

In both sexes, infertility can be caused by hypogonadism and disorders of sexual determination and sexual differentiation where a role may be played either by hormonal secretion or receptor response.

In women, genetic factors have an impact on the number and quality of oocytes, and besides chromosomal defects and fragile X syndrome they also include genetic disorders of oocyte maturation [11], endometriosis [12,13], polycystic ovarian syndrome, BRCA1/2 gene mutations, and ZP2 and ZP3 gene mutations [14]. In addition, genetic causes of implantation disorders, lethal genetic mutations [15,16], and endometrial receptivity disorders occur where an important role is played, in particular, by the progesterone receptor A and estrogen receptor beta. Causes of infertility also include genetic causes of recurrent abortion, such as the HLA-C and HLA-G status, and numerous other genes 1.7 men, genetic causes of infertility account for up to 30% of cases [17]. They include chromosomal defects (Klinefelter syndrome, Down syndrome, chromosomal rearrangements). Deletions in the region of AZFa, AZFb, or AZFc are one of the most common causes of nonobstructive azoospermia and severe oligozoospermia. Additional causes include mutations and polymorphisms in genes for the receptors for FSH, LH, and androgens, in the genes CFTR, AURKC, PICK1, SPATA16, CFAP43, CFAP44, SEPT12, CATSPER, ADAM2, PLCZ1, and others [18,19].

Genetic disorders can lead to various syndromes, including fertility disorders and disorders of the structure or function of other organs [20]. Genetically related motility disorders of the cilia and flagella are typical cases; on the one hand, these disorders are associated with impaired sperm motility, and on the other with impaired respiratory tract function. For example, they include Kartagener syndrome, also called ciliary dyskinesia syndrome with autosomal recessive inheritance. Various organs of the mucociliary transport are affected, e.g., the bronchi with bronchiectases; the sperm becomes immotile due to flagellar pathology; polyps form in paranasal sinuses. Situs viscerum inversus may be another characteristic. No routine diagnostic procedures have yet been widely used for this syndrome.

Another group is represented by mutations in the androgen receptor gene where, besides reproductive disorders, neurological diseases are present. A relationship is known not only between CFTR gene mutations and male infertility, but also between autosomal dominant polycystic kidney or kidney agenesis and ejaculate parameters.

In male fertility disorders, 46,XY gonadal dysgenesis, anorchia, cerebello-oculo-renal syndrome, and hypospadias are more common in the offspring.

Known genetic disorders with a negative impact on female fertility, associated with the risk of transferring other diseases, include, e.g., fragile X syndrome and BRCA1/2 gene mutations.

The clinical team at Repromeda offer the PANDA test to help patients better understand and manage the genetic risks of reproduction as well as adding information and elucidation of some potential factors that may cause or impact fertility or the patients' chance of success following IVF procedures. This test is on the cutting edge of medical treatment, not only in the fertility field but in medicine in general.

Genetic Testing of Gamete Donors

Genetic testing of gamete donors plays a substantial role in reproductive medicine. The effort is to exclude the transfer of serious genetic defects to the offspring of gamete donation recipients. Besides the medical point of view, a role is also played by legal regulation and the potential forensic consequences of giving birth to a child with a congenital defect.

As a rule, a general framework for genetic testing of donors is given by legal regulations and national standards. Currently, as mentioned previously, the spectrum of genetic tests required in various countries differs and most commonly includes testing of the karyotype and carrier status of recessive gene mutations for the given population, specifically those for cystic fibrosis, spinal muscular atrophy, and congenital deafness (connexin 26). Other tested mutations are optional and based on the opinion of a particular site.

Obviously, many more recessive hereditary diseases exist besides the three selected and regularly tested ones; on the other hand, the carrier status of these and a number of other diseases is relatively common in the population, and therefore it is very difficult in practice to select donors with no carrier status of the growing number of tested recessive mutations. In addition, the tendency to exclude any mutation carrier status from the population does not seem meaningful from any point of view. Therefore, genetic "matching" of donors and recipients in the event of an acceptable residual risk seems to be an effective solution [5,21]. The task of professional associations is to develop appropriate guidelines in the near future for the matching rules of reproductive material donors for the case of non-partner donation. The use of ECS in third-party reproduction is currently developing faster than most clinicians and patients might be able to keep up with. *It is imperative that clinicians, technologists, and others involved in assisted reproduction continue to develop education around the genetics of fertility and infertility.*

Therapeutic Procedures for Fertility Disorders and Genetic Defect Risks Using Genetic Methods

The genetic status of the embryo is one of the essential properties that affects its implantation, the successful course of pregnancy, and the probability of giving birth to a healthy child. Most aneuploid embryos are lost in the preimplantation period or in the first trimester of pregnancy; alternatively, in the event of so-called birthable defects they may result in the birth of a defective child. Structural chromosomal defects lead to reduced fertility and entail the risk of giving birth to a child with a congenital defect as a result of unbalanced chromosomal rearrangement. Gene mutations may lead to a child with so-called monogenic disease. The entirety of these problems is managed through PGT.

Nowadays, the benefit of PGT of monogenic diseases (PGT-M) and structural chromosomal defects (PGT-SR) is generally recognized [22–25]. Various technologies are used for these purposes by sites, including karyomapping as the most universal and flexible method functioning on the principle of SNP genotyping. The resolution of this method for testing amplified DNA from blastocyst trophectoderm ranges from approximately 10 Mb.

Based on SNP data analysis of the parents and of a reference with a known or properly determined/derived genotype, karyomapping [26] allows indirect DNA diagnosis of genetic patterns showing Mendelian inheritance. The method provides reliable simultaneous detection of haploidy, triploidy, monosomy, meiotic trisomy, uniparental disomy, partial chromosomal loss (>10 Mb), and mosaicism. The method allows limited detection of trisomy of mitotic origin and partial chromosomal gains. Based on SNP data, karyomapping detects contamination, determines allelic dropout (ADO) in the tested embryos, and also verifies parental status and any relation of the reference to the tested embryos. In addition, the method allows two and more mutations of imbalances to be detected at the same time. Karyomapping is covered in several subsequent chapters of this book.

PGT-A

Surprisingly, discussion of the benefit and effectiveness of PGT-A, whose main purpose is to increase the success rate of assisted reproduction, can still be encountered in some forums [27]. The effects of PGT-A include, but are not limited to, reduced failure rate of implantation, reduced rate of spontaneous abortion, and financial savings [22,27,28]. Although PGT-A opponents call for further randomized studies in the framework of evidence-based medicine, PGT-A supporters argue that not performing PGT-A, particularly in indicated groups (the age factor, recurrent pregnancy losses, the male-meiotic factor, status post chemotherapy/actinotherapy, etc.), can no longer be viewed as ethical given that positive effects already follow from retrospective studies and the evaluation of results of national registries of assisted reproduction (e.g., in the United States). The author believes that PGT-A should be a routine and in modern reproductive medicine an indispensable part of infertility therapy using IVF methods.

The MPS method is currently the predominant method for PGT-A [29]. MPS allows the testing of aneuploidy of all human chromosomes, detects unbalanced chromosomal aberrations sized >15 Mb, and can detect triploid embryos 69,XXY and 69,XYY. In addition, this method detects mosaicism in trophectoderm samples in the range of 30%–80%. MPS cannot detect haploid chromosomal sets, triploidy 69,XXX, tetraploidy and balanced chromosomal rearrangements in trophectoderm samples. The reliability of genetic testing of non-mosaicism trophectoderm samples is estimated as >99.5%.

Certainly, scientific evidence continues to mount on the usefulness of PGT-A clinically. Speaking to patients about PGT-A takes up a large amount of time in the clinical conversation ahead of and after an IVF cycle. Helping patients understand the pros and cons of testing embryos during IVF and aiding in their decision-making around genetic testing can be time-consuming for everyone involved in the process.

Mosaicism

The phenomenon of mosaicism has emerged in the issue of PGT-A with the onset of the aforementioned modern technologies based on MPS that support a high resolution of the CNVs on the whole-chromosome and subchromosomal levels (segmental aneuploidy). Primarily, it is a biological phenomenon naturally present in the early stage of embryonic cell division, whose rate decreases with the development of the embryo to the blastocyst stage. Based on current knowledge, PGT in blastomeres of an embryo approximately 3 days old must be viewed as professionally unacceptable and non-lege artis. The method of choice consists of trophectoderm biopsy from the blastocyst on day 5–7 of embryonic development with subsequent vitrification of the biopsied embryos [30]. The purpose is to subsequently choose one euploid embryo for transfer to the endometrium in a non-stimulated cycle (either using the natural ovulation cycle or HRT cycle). The best results are achieved if the embryo is chosen based on combined criteria according to the PGT-A result and semi-continuous monitoring using the time-lapse method.

However, due to the characteristics of their reproductive cells, not all couples can obtain an optimal embryo, i.e., one that is euploid and morphologically and morphokinetically optimal. Only mosaic embryos are available to choose from in many couples. Given that information in the literature confirms the possibility of giving birth to healthy children after the transfer of mosaic embryos [31], great attention should be paid to this issue [3]. When it is unlikely that a couple will have euploid embryos or if the couple does not wish to undergo any further IVF cycles for various reasons and wants the transfer of a mosaic embryo, they should be given this option after a detailed consultation and thorough counseling by the reproductologist and clinical geneticist. The consultation should also include the determination of preference of a specific mosaic embryo, provided that more such embryos exist. The chance of giving birth to a healthy child depends on the ratio of healthy and aneuploid cells and on the particular chromosome or locus involved. Embryos without a mosaic in risk chromosomes related to birthable defects (chromosomes X, 13, 18, 21) or without excessive (high-percentage) and complex mosaics (PGDIS Position Statement) [32] should be prioritized. The transfer of a mosaic embryo can be expected to be associated with an implantation rate decreased 2–3 times and an abortion rate increased 2–3 times. In the case of ongoing pregnancy, invasive prenatal diagnosis is recommended. In this respect, PGT-A should rather be understood as a method that determines the optimal rank of embryos according to the expected success rate achievable after the transfer and not only as a method to exclude the transfer of aneuploid embryos

[33]. As mentioned previously, an optimal success rate can be achieved based on summation of the results of semi-continuous embryonic monitoring using the time-lapse system and of the PGT-A results. Other chapters in this book deal extensively with PGT-A, mosaicism, and transfer of mosaic embryos.

Genetic Methods to Detect the Window of Implantation

Genetic and morphological quality of the embryo is necessary to induce pregnancy; however, with no receptive endometrium this is insufficient to achieve successful assisted reproduction. The list of genetic tests done in modern reproductive medicine should also include gene expression testing, based on which the window of implantation is determined (personalized window of implantation [pWOI] [34]). In 2009, Igenomix patented the ERA® (Endometrial Receptivity Analysis) test; this test has been converted to the NGS platform, and in connection with bioinformatics technologies it allows detection of the expression of 248 genes on the mRNA level. The test identifies the receptive, pre-receptive, and post-receptive phase with high reliability, and thus it has become a good-quality predictor of the window of implantation. Genetic testing has been clearly demonstrated to be superior to histological endometrial classification [35] as described by Noyes et al. in 1975 [36]. As demonstrated by data in the literature, the determined window of implantation remains constant in individual women for 29–40 months.

The importance of the ERA test lies in its capability to determine an individual window of implantation with accuracy, and to increase the chance of successful implantation upon subsequent personalized embryo transfer [37].

Genetic Testing in the Surrogacy Program

Certain specific aspects of the surrogacy program should be mentioned, where good-quality genetic testing is highly desirable. Although the uterine factor seems to be a major problem in couples requesting surrogacy, it should be taken into account that combined factors are present in such couples, very commonly including advanced reproductive age. According to European law, the mother is the woman who gives birth to the child, and therefore also if the developing fetus is genetically defective, only the mother can decide to terminate the pregnancy—in this case solely the surrogate mother, and the intended (biological) parents have no possibility of intervening in this process with their own will. Therefore, it is recommended to perform high-quality and detailed pre-therapeutic genetic testing in the reproductive partners, and subsequently to perform PGT-A in the embryos to reduce the genetic risk.

Cases where the woman has a congenital uterine defect, for example, Mayer–Rokitanski–Küster–Hauser (MRKH) syndrome, represent another group of couples where genetic counseling should play a significant role. These women can often use their own oocytes for fertilization; in this case they should be informed about the risk of transferring the congenital defect to the next generation. The most common mutations associated with the MRKH syndrome include deletions in the 17q12 region containing the genes TCF2 and LHX1 [38–40]. Heterozygous mutations of TCF2 were initially associated with MODY5 syndrome with malformations of the kidneys and their impaired function. A subgroup of female patients with heterozygous mutations of TCF2 had malformations of the reproductive tract, such as uterus bicornis, uterus didelphys, and aplasia of Müllerian duct, as well as renal defects with the absence of diabetes [41,42]. This indicates an important role of the TCF2 gene in the formation of the urogenital tract. MRKH syndrome has also been associated with five heterozygous mutations in LHX1 gene [43–45]. Partial duplication of the SHOX gene was found in an unaffected father and two daughters with MRKH syndrome type I [46].

Considering the fact that previously this was an unsolvable cause of infertility, no process of routine genetic diagnosis has been developed for these syndromes. However, the increasing demand for surrogacy in these couples should stimulate clinical as well as molecular genetics to thoroughly explore the specific type of heredity and mutations of candidate genes associated with MRKH syndromes and with other defects in order to offer targeted PGT-M and thus to prevent the inheritance of these developmental defects, serious for reproduction.

Genetic Methods in the Control of Therapeutic Results

If needed, feedback on therapeutic results can be provided by prenatal follow-up assessments using invasive or noninvasive methods. Such tests should be used where there are factors with an impact on test sensitivity or specificity, including, e.g., the transfer of mosaic embryos. Noninvasive prenatal testing (NIPT) is based on the presence of free fetal DNA released from apoptotic placental cells in the mother's blood [47]. Currently, in cases of mosaic embryo transfers, it is universally recommended to use invasive methods; however, future use of noninvasive tests is not unthinkable with the increasing robustness and accuracy of NIPT methods.

The testing of chorionic villi from abortion materials is another type of assessment; this testing makes it possible to verify previous preimplantation testing and to validate laboratory methods. More than 70% of the findings in spontaneous abortions samples are aneuploid [48], and the method allows an evaluation of reliability of the diagnosis by comparing the results in abortions of pregnancies with and without the use of PGT.

Summary

Genetic testing is an inseparable part of reproductive medicine and its need is naturally increasing in connection with requirements for higher quality and safety of the therapy. It not only helps to improve the accuracy of the diagnosis, target and personalize the therapy, and thus achieve success in the shortest time possible, but it also provides financial savings to the healthcare system and to the patient. The essential pillars of current genetic testing before inclusion in an *in vitro* fertilization program, both on the part of the reproductive partners and/or the donors, include karyotyping and molecular genetic analysis performed if possible in multiple-gene panels. Genetic tests included in these panels should be rationally considered and chosen in such a way that their results can have a positive impact on the therapy and minimize the transfer of a genetic risk to the next generation. Generally, the higher the number of mutations included in the panel, the higher the proportion of variants—of unclear meaning at the given moment—assessed by the test. Also, the ethical risks associated with coincidental findings should always be taken into account as well as the fact that although extended testing substantially decreases the risk of an inherited disease in the next generation, it can never eliminate such a risk completely. Information on the benign nature or pathogenicity of individual mutations/variants may change with the increasing scope of experience. Targeted PGT-M should be recommended as the first choice in the partner donation program when a genetic risk of transferring a hereditary disease is captured. In case of non-partner donation, matching of a suitable donor is the solution, excluding the mutation carried by the recipient with an acceptable residual risk.

PGT of embryos has become an integral part of assisted reproduction and it helps a healthy child to be conceived even in couples for whom this was not possible in the past. Regarding PGT-A, requirements to increase the probability of embryo implantation come to the fore, while reducing the risk of abortion, and last but not least, to rank the embryos according to the expected success rate, in connection with embryo morphology evaluation using the time-lapse system. As to the real chance of giving birth to a healthy child even after the transfer of a mosaic embryo, reproductive specialists and clinical geneticists should become acquainted with an optimal strategy for mosaic embryo transfer and be able to inform the partners about the relevant data and provide the support necessary for them to make a free decision.

Modern reproductive medicine also includes the detection of the window of implantation into the endometrium using gene expression and subsequent personalization of the transfer with respect to the determined result.

In the years to come, we can expect a further steep rise in the knowledge of genetics and genomics, which will lead to further development of genetic diagnosis, not only in reproductive medicine. Massive development can be expected in the segment of noninvasive tests, which, thanks to increasing accuracy, will very probably compete with invasive tests.

REFERENCES

1. Evans HJ, Buckton KE, Sumner AT. Cytological mapping or human chromosomes-results obtained with quinacrine fluorescence and the acetic-saline-Giemsa techniques. *Chromosoma.* 1971;35:310–25.
2. Grant SF et al. SNP genotyping on a genome-wide amplified DOP-PCR template. *Nucleic Acids Res.* 2002;30:e125.
3. Harper JC et al. On behalf of the European Society of Human Reproduction and Embryology and European Society of Human Genetics. Recent developments in genetics and medically assisted reproduction: From research to clinical applications. *Europ J Human Genet.* 2018;26:12–33.
4. Patel B et al. Comprehensive genetic testing for female and male infertility using next-generation sequencing. *J Assist Reprod Genet.* 2018;35:1489–96.
5. Abulí A et al. NGS-based assay for the identification of individuals carrying recessive genetic mutations in reproductive medicine. *Hum Mutat.* 2016;37:516–23.
6. Henneman L et al. Responsible implementation of expanded carrier screening. *Eur J Hum Genet.* 2016;24:e1–12.
7. Frampton GM et al. Development and validation of a clinical cancer genomic profiling test based on massively parallel DNA sequencing. *Nat Biotechnol [Internet].* 2013;31:1023–31.
8. Celestino-Soper PBS et al. Validation and utilization of a clinical next-generation sequencing panel for selected cardiovascular disorders. *Front Cardiovasc Med [Internet].* 2017;4:1–11.
9. Oliveira KC et al. Prevalence of the polymorphism MTHFR A1298C and not MTHFR C677 T is related to chromosomal aneuploidy in Brazilian Turner Syndrome patients. *Arq Bras Endocrinol Metabol.* 2008;52(8):1374–81.
10. Mallepaly R, Butler PR, Herati AS, Lamb DJ. Genetic basis of male and female infertility. *Monogr Hum Genet.* 2017;21:1–16.
11. Zheng H et al. Application of next generation sequencing for 24-chromosome aneuploidy screening of human preimplantation embryos. *Mol Cytogenet.* 2015;8(38):1–9.
12. Borghese B et al. Recent insights on the genetics and epigenetics of endometriosis. *Clin Genet.* 2017;91:254–64.
13. Matalliotakis M et al. The role of gene polymorphisms in endometriosis. *Mol Med Rep.* 2017;6(5):5881–6.
14. Liu W et al. Dosage effects of ZP2 and ZP3 heterozygous mutations cause human infertility. *Hum Genet.* 2017;136(8):975–85.
15. Alazami AM et al. TLE6 mutation causes the earliest known human embryonic lethality. *Genome Biol.* 2015;16(240):1–8.
16. Yanez LZ et al. Human oocyte developmental potential is predicted by mechanical properties within hours after fertilization. *Nat Commun.* 2016;7(10809):1–12.
17. Neto FTL et al. Genetics of male infertility. *Curr Urol Rep [Internet].* 2016;17:70–82.
18. Mitchell MJ et al. Single gene defects leading to sperm quantitative anomalies. *Clin Genet.* 2017;91(2):208–16.
19. Ray PF et al. Genetic abnormalities leading to qualitative defects of sperm morphology or function. *Clin Genet.* 2017;91(2):217–32.
20. Tarín JJ et al. Infertility etiologies are genetically and clinically linked with other diseases in single meta-diseases. *Reprod Biol Endocrinol.* 2015;13(31):1–11.
21. Dondorp W et al. ESHRE Task Force on Ethics and Law 21: Genetic screening of gamete donors: Ethical issues. *Hum Reprod.* 2014;29:1353–9.
22. Sermon K et al. The why, the how and the when of PGS 2.0: Current practices and expert opinions of fertility specialists, molecular biologists, and embryologists. *Mol Hum Reprod.* 2016;22:845–57.
23. Thornhill AR et al. Karyomapping-a comprehensive means of simultaneous monogenic and cytogenetic PGD: Comparison with standard approaches in real time for Marfan syndrome. *J Assist Reprod Genet.* 2015;32:347–56.
24. Vermeesch JR, Voet T, Devriendt K. Prenatal and preimplantation genetic diagnosis. *Nat Rev Genet.* 2016;17:643–56.
25. Zamani Esteki M et al. Concurrent whole-genome haplotyping and copy-number profiling of single cells. *Am J Hum Genet.* 2015;96:894–912.
26. Handyside AH et al. Karyomapping: A universal method for genome wide analysis of genetic disease based on mapping crossovers between parental haplotypes. *J Med Genet.* 2010;47(10):651–8.

27. Geraedts J, Sermon K. Preimplantation genetic screening 2.0: The theory. *Mol Hum Reprod.* 2016;22:839–44.

28. Munné S, Cohen J. Advanced maternal age patients benefit from preimplantation genetic diagnosis of aneuploidy. *Fertil Steril.* 2017;107(5):1145–6.

29. Wells D. Next-generation sequencing: The dawn of a new era for preimplantation genetic diagnostics. *Fertil Steril.* 2014;101:1250–1.

30. Coates A et al. Optimal euploid embryo transfer strategy, fresh versus frozen, after preimplantation genetic screening with next generation sequencing: A randomized controlled trial. *Fertil Steril.* 2017;07(3):723–30.

31. Greco E, Minasi MG, Fiorentino F. Healthy babies after intrauterine transfer of mosaic aneuploid blastocysts. *N Engl J Med.* 2015;373:2089–90.

32. Cram DS et al. Position Statement on the Transfer of Mosaic Embryos 2019. *Reprod Biomed Online.* 2019;39(Suppl 1):e1–4.

33. Maxwell SM et al. Why do euploid embryos miscarry? A case-control study comparing the rate of aneuploidy within presumed euploid embryos that resulted in miscarriage or live birth using next-generation sequencing. *Fertil Steril.* 2016;106:1414–9.

34. Díaz-Gimeno P et al. A genomic diagnostic tool for human endometrial receptivity based on the transcriptomic signature. *Fertil Steril.* 2011;95(1):50–60.

35. Díaz-Gimeno P et al. The accuracy and reproducibility of the endometrial receptivity array is superior to histology as a diagnostic method for endometrial receptivity. *Fertil Steril.* 2013;99(2):508–17.

36. Noyes RW, Hertig AT, Rock J. Dating the endometrial biopsy. *Am J Obstet Gynecol.* 1975;122(2):262–3.

37. Garrido-Gómez T et al. Profiling the gene signature of endometrial receptivity: Clinical results. *Fertil Steril.* 2013;99(4):1078–85.

38. Bernardini L et al. Recurrent microdeletion at 17q12 as a cause of Mayer-Rokitansky-Kuster-Hauser (MRKH) syndrome: Two case reports. *Orphanet J Rare Dis.* 2009;25:1–6.

39. Coffinier C, Barra J, Babinet C, Yaniv M. Expression of the vHNF1/HNF1beta homeoprotein gene during mouse organogenesis. *Mech Dev.* 1999;89:211–3.

40. Kolatsi-Joannou M et al. Hepatocyte nuclear factor-1beta: A new kindred with renal cysts and diabetes and gene expression in normal human development. *J Am Soc Nephrol.* 2001;12:2175–80.

41. Bingham C et al. Solitary functioning kidney and diverse genital tract malformations associated with hepatocyte nuclear factor-1beta mutations. *Kidney Int.* 2002;61:1243–51.

42. Lindner TH et al. A novel syndrome of diabetes mellitus, renal dysfunction and genital malformation associated with a partial deletion of the pseudo-POU domain of hepatocyte nuclear factor-1beta. *Hum Mol Genet.* 1999;8:2001–8.

43. Ledig S et al. Frame shift mutation of LHX1 is associated with Mayer-Rokitansky-Kuster-Hauser (MRKH) syndrome. *Hum Reprod.* 2012;27:2872–5.

44. Ledig S et al. Recurrent aberrations identified by array-CGH in patients with Mayer-Rokitansky-Kuster-Hauser syndrome. *Fertil Steril.* 2011;95:589–1594.

45. Sandbacka M et al. TBX6, LHX1 and copy number variations in the complex genetics of Mullerian aplasia. *Orphanet J Rare Dis.* 2013;8:125.

46. Gervasini C et al. SHOX duplications found in some cases with type I Mayer-Rokitansky-Kuster-Hauser syndrome. *Genet Med.* 2010;12(10):634–40.

47. Lo YMD et al. Presence of fetal DNA in maternal plasma and serum. *Lancet.* 1997;350:485–7.

48. Soler A et al. Overview of chromosome abnormalities in first trimester miscarriages: A series of 1,011 consecutive chorionic villi sample karyotypes. *Cytogenet Genome Res.* 2017;152(2):81–9.

2

Genetic Counseling for Preimplantation Genetic Testing

Lauri D. Black and Jill M. Fischer

CONTENTS

Introduction

Genetic counselors are Masters-level healthcare professionals with advanced training in medical genetics and counseling. These professionals specialize in the analysis of medical and family history information to formulate a genetic risk assessment. They educate patients and other members of the patient's healthcare team about genetic disorders and their inheritance patterns. They help guide patients in making well-informed decisions about the screening and diagnostic testing options that are most congruent with the patient's values and goals based on their specific medical and family history. Genetic counselors work in an assortment of settings including university medical centers, private medical offices, diagnostic and research laboratories, health maintenance organizations, government agencies, advocacy groups or not-for-profit organizations, and in private practice. Areas of practice include preconception/prenatal, pediatric, adult, and general genetics care. There are growing numbers of specialties, such as cancer, neurology, cardiology, ophthalmology, dermatology, psychiatry, and infertility/assisted reproductive technologies, pharmacogenomics, precision medicine and disease specific clinics. With the expanding utilization of preimplantation genetic testing (PGT), genetic counselors are increasingly becoming part of the reproductive medicine healthcare team. This chapter focuses on the training and practice of genetic counselors in the United States, where the field has historically been more commonly incorporated into healthcare, but has wider implications for the practice of genetic counseling in other countries.

Training, Certification, and Licensure

Although a relative newcomer to the field of healthcare, the addition of genetic counselors to the workforce has been rapidly expanding since the inception of the very first training program at Sarah Lawrence

College in Bronxville, New York in 1969. As the profession grew and genetic counselors gained a unique identity in healthcare, the need for a professional organization was born. The National Society of Genetic Counselors (NSGC) was therefore incorporated in 1979 [1]. In the brief 47 years since the first class of genetic counselors graduated, the demand for genetic counselors has dramatically grown. On June 1, 2018, CareerCast.com released its Jobs Rated Report listing Genetic Counseling as the number 1 rated job for 2018 [2]. In 2017 and 2018, the *U.S. News and World Report* named genetic counseling as one of the "25 Amazing Health Care Support Jobs" [3,4]. The Bureau of Labor Statistics predicts employment as a genetic counselor to grow 29% between 2016 and 2026 compared to average growth of 7% across all occupations [5]. This statistic ranks the occupation of genetic counseling as 14th on a list of fastest growing occupations in the United States [5]. This growth is likely spurred by the U.S. Supreme Court ruling against patenting of genes in 2013 and the National Institutes of Health's Precision Medicine Initiative [6–8]. This environment opened the market to an increase in genetic test providers and promoted less expensive methods of genetic analysis. Such circumstances also allow for the expansion of research into the genetic etiologies of disease and how genetic variation interplays with nongenetic factors to cause disease, fueling advances in precision medicine. This expansion requires a medical professional who not only understands the science, but who is also capable of navigating the psychosocial, ethical, and legal aspects of such; thus the increase in demand for genetic counselors.

For this profession, the Masters in Genetic Counseling is a terminal degree. The degree program is cohort based, starting each fall semester lasting a minimum of 21 months or 2 academic years. The curriculum includes education in the didactic, clinical, and research arenas. Training programs in North America must be approved and certified by the Accreditation Council for Genetic Counseling (ACGC) [9]. As of 2018, the ACGC has conferred full accreditation status to 30 genetic counseling training programs, with another 11 being granted new program accreditation status in the United States alone [10]. Additionally, there are four training programs in Canada, three with full accreditation and one with new program accreditation [10]. Worldwide, there are an additional eight programs in Europe, five in Asia, two in Australia and New Zealand, two in the Middle East, two in Africa, and one in Central/South America [11].

Upon graduation from an accredited program, students will be eligible to sit for the professional certification exam from the American Board of Genetic Counseling (ABGC) [12]. Passing the exam confers the status of Certified Genetic Counselor (CGC) and enables the individual to obtain licensure if one's state of employment requires such [13]. Licensed genetic counselors can use the designations of LCGC or LGC [14]. Both certification and licensure are time limited. Recertification is done every 5 years via continuing education units (CEUs) or retaking of the exam [15]. Licenses must be renewed on a regular basis as per each state's requirements. Currently, about half of all states require licensure to practice as a genetic counselor, though this number increases annually (Figure 2.1) [16].

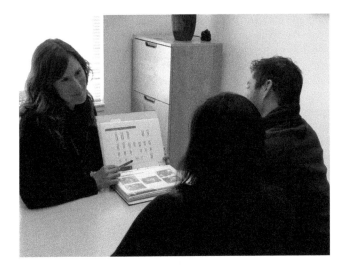

FIGURE 2.1 A typical genetic counseling session.

Definition, Process, and Principles of Genetic Counseling

The NSGC defines genetic counseling as the process of helping people understand and adapt to the medical, psychological, and familial implications of genetic contributions to disease [17]. It further defines this process by stating that it integrates (1) collection and interpretation of family and medical histories to assess the chance of disease occurrence or recurrence; (2) education about inheritance, testing, management, prevention, resources, and research; and (3) counseling to promote informed choices and adaptation to the risk or condition [17].

The genetic counseling process is based on two main principles: non-directiveness and patient autonomy [17]. The NSGC explains that "genetic counselors can help incorporate the latest genetic science into the healthcare team by providing comprehensive genetic services to patients," and that genetic counselors "advanced training in counseling helps provide the emotional support patients need as complex genetic information is translated into sometimes-difficult healthcare decisions" [18]. A key tenet of genetic counseling is to provide education and psychosocial support to patients and their families through in a non-directive fashion. As the profession has evolved, the idea of "non-directive" genetic counseling has morphed into an ethos of fostering optimal patient care by providing balanced information, refraining from imposing the counselor's own values on their patients' decisions, and guiding patients, through psychosocial support, to the decision they feel is right for them [19]. In this way, genetic counseling differs significantly from more the prescriptive approach taken in most other fields of medicine. In essence, the genetic counselor educates and supports patients to make the best available decision for themselves and their families rather than instructing the patient about the "correct" course of action.

Main Components of Genetic Counseling for PGT

In assisted reproductive technologies (ART), PGT genetic counselors typically work either in the laboratory that provides the embryo testing or with the *in vitro* fertilization (IVF) center that conducts the cycle, and creates and biopsies the embryos. Though roles of the genetic counselor in these two settings can differ, ideally those in either setting provide comprehensive care as outlined previously. A basic difference in the consult between the PGT laboratory and IVF center genetic counselor is the service delivery model. Given the PGT laboratory is typically not a part of the IVF center and therefore can be in a different state or even country from the IVF group and patient, the genetic consult is typically conducted by telephone. For genetic counselors at the IVF center, communication with the patients can be done via phone or video conferencing, but consults are usually conducted face-to-face. Other differences will be highlighted throughout this chapter. This chapter discusses most common test techniques and focuses on genetic counseling best practices.

It is possible that the initial discussion of PGT will be with a genetic counselor outside of an ART setting, such as in a pediatric, prenatal, or cancer setting. In this case, this genetic counselor may serve as a referral source for the ART clinic and PGT laboratory. The ART/PGT genetic counselor will then serve as a case manager as it pertains to genetic testing services.

Genetic counseling for PGT can be subdivided into pretest and post-test counseling. In the pretest consultation, medical and family histories are obtained and formulated into a pedigree. There is discussion of risks associated with the indication for testing, the safety of embryo biopsy [20], all viable test options for this indication (preimplantation, prenatal, and postnatal), and means of mitigating the risk (patients' use of own gametes, donor gametes, and adoption) as appropriate. The benefits, risks, and limitations of such test options are also discussed in detail to promote informed decision-making. Follow-up prenatal testing recommendations after PGT are discussed. Any additional patient or family member testing as indicated by the medical and family histories is discussed. The genetic counselor in the IVF center may coordinate such testing, whereas the genetic counselor in the PGT laboratory will recommend such testing be performed through the referring IVF center or other provider. Additionally, psychosocial support and other resources may be provided as needed. If the genetic counselor is affiliated with an IVF clinic, then discussion of clinic specific outcomes, such as implantation, pregnancy, and livebirth rates, is appropriate.

Typically, a summary letter is generated by the PGT lab genetic counselor to document the details of the consultation and provided for patient and referring physician use. The American Society of Reproductive Medicine (ASRM) also recommends that each clinic's policies on transfer of embryos that test positive be reviewed with patients in advance of testing [21].

During post-test counseling, test results are reviewed in detail. Frequently, there is a repeat of the discussion of limitations of testing as well as the definition of what constitutes a "normal" result, and the specifics of any abnormalities detected. If the discussion is being led by an IVF clinic based genetic counselor, then clinic policies on transfer or long-term storage of embryos with positive results is also reviewed. Additionally, if an embryo or embryos are transferred, once again reviewing options for prenatal and postnatal confirmatory testing is appropriate. Of note, post-test counseling may be handled differently by the PGT laboratory. Given the PGT laboratory is not always privy to quality or quantity of embryos after biopsy, most PGT laboratories report the PGT results directly to the referring physician or IVF center, not the patient. Genetic counselors at the PGT laboratory therefore conduct a post-test results discussion with the referring physician per request and will discuss results with the patient if directed to do so by the referring physician. Discussion of predictability for subsequent cycles and additional future options is usually done with patient after IVF/PGT cycle failure.

Genetic Counseling for Preimplantation Genetic Testing

PGT for Aneuploidy (PGT-A)

Aneuploidy has long been recognized as a significant reproductive genetic risk, independent of family history, and having a strong correlation with maternal age. Addressing aneuploidy risk has been the focus of many prenatal testing options for decades. Given many IVF patients are of "advanced maternal age," this focus has also expanded to PGT. It is therefore not surprising that aneuploidy screening has become a common reason for PGT [20,22].

Since the advent of PGT-A, there have been significant changes in test technology that have allowed for improvements in comprehensiveness, accuracy, and now resolution (Figure 2.2).

Initially, aneuploidy screening was performed on polar bodies or individual blastomeres biopsied from cleavage-stage (day 3) embryos using fluorescence *in-situ* hybridization (FISH) probes for select chromosomes. Initially only the sex chromosomes, X and Y, were tested, but later use of sequential hybridization of multicolor probe panels allowed for up to 12 chromosomes to be tested. In counseling

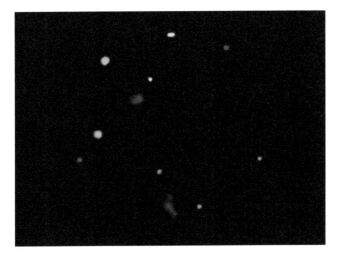

FIGURE 2.2   Images of five-probe FISH showing three green fluorescent probes corresponding to trisomy 21. (Courtesy of Jill Fischer, Reprogenetics.)

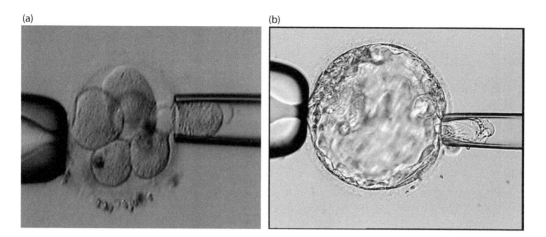

FIGURE 2.3   (a), cleavage-stage (day 3) single-cell (blastomere) biopsy. (b), multiple cell trophectoderm biopsy of a blastocyst. (Courtesy of Jill Fischer, Reprogenetics.)

about limitations, it was essential to outline not only the cumulative detection/error rate based on the number of probes being used but also that not all chromosomes were being evaluated.

While cleavage-stage biopsy is still more common in some countries, in the United States, where PGT is more frequently performed, the standard is now trophectoderm biopsy of blastocyst-stage (day 5, 6, or, less commonly, 7) embryos (Figure 2.3).

As the goal was to test for all 24 chromosomes, molecular-based tests of array comparative genomic hybridization (aCGH) and single-nucleotide polymorphism (SNP) array supplanted FISH once able to be applied to single cells. This shift toward testing all chromosome pairs with chromosomal microarray platforms led some early adopters to term such testing "comprehensive chromosome screening" ("CCS") to distinguish it from the limited chromosome screening ability of FISH. These microarrays had higher detection rates and lower error rates than multiple-probe FISH [22,23]. There was considerable controversy surrounding the clinical benefit of aneuploidy screening of cleavage-stage biopsy with FISH that carried over into the initial years of utilizing blastocyst biopsy with microarrays (see subsequent chapters). However, data began emerging that demonstrated improved clinical outcomes after aneuploidy screening with blastocyst biopsy and microarrays (Figure 2.4) [22].

More recently, aneuploidy screening methodology has transitioned to next-generation sequencing (NGS) platforms. At the time of writing, this is the most common test platform used in major PGT labs in the United States. Among other potential benefits, there is higher resolution with NGS and

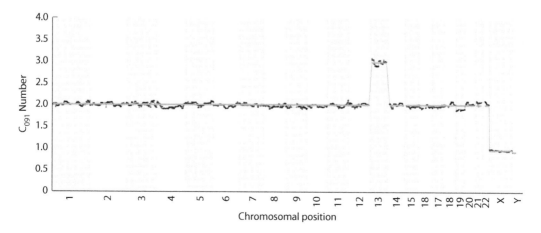

FIGURE 2.4   MiSEquation NGS platform result of 47,XY,+13. (Courtesy of G. Harton.)

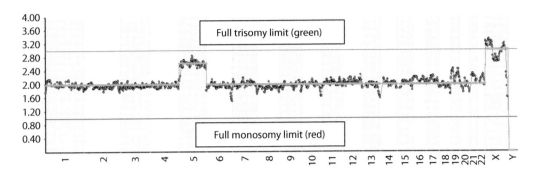

FIGURE 2.5 PGT-A via NGS revealing mosaic results. Results are below full trisomy limit and indicate ~80% mosaicism for trisomy 5 in sample. (Courtesy of Jill Fischer, Reprogenetics.)

a greater ability to detect smaller segments of chromosomes that might be deleted (missing) or duplicated (added), sometimes called segmental aneuploidy. NGS also allows for clearer detection and optional reporting of aneuploidy mosaicism within a sample of biopsied cells compared to microarrays (Figure 2.5) [24].

The pretest PGT-A genetics consult includes the components outlined previously. Two topics of discussion which differ from prenatal aneuploidy consults are aneuploidy rates and mosaicism. Aneuploidy rates in embryos are dramatically higher than those seen in pregnancy. The advanced maternal age patient who would be given a 1%–2% chance of aneuploidy at time of amniocentesis would be informed that a majority of embryos will be aneuploid (Table 2.1). The genetic counselor therefore must explain that the chronological stage at time of testing dictates the rate of aneuploidy, with highest rates being in the preimplantation stage. Rates drop as a pregnancy continues from first trimester to delivery given that most aneuploid pregnancies result in loss.

Embryo mosaicism has historically been discussed as a potential limitation in interpretation of PGT results or with discrepancies between preimplantation and pre- or postnatal aneuploidy test results. However, it has not been until the advent of NGS-based PGT-A that the possibility of counseling about mosaicism identified in a biopsy sample has become a consideration. There are varied opinions and much discussion about how to manage mosaic results.

Counseling for mosaic aneuploid results is currently complicated by the relative paucity of prenatal and postnatal outcome data after mosaic embryo transfer. Statements have been published by professional organizations [25,26] and continue to evolve as more data become available. However, it is recognized that there is still much to learn before confident counseling of expected outcomes is possible. Genetic counselors are well suited and specifically trained to relay this type of complex and ambiguous information to patients and help them navigate decision making.

It is important to underscore that PGT results reflect the sample itself. Therefore, while NGS for aneuploidy may be able to detect mosaicism in a biopsy sample, it can neither diagnose nor rule out mosaicism in the whole embryo (Figure 2.6).

TABLE 2.1

Aneuploidy Rates in Embryos

Maternal Age	Aneuploidy Rate (%)
<35	38
35–37	47
38–40	62
41–42	77
>42	85

Source: From Reprogenetics data. (Courtesy of Jill Fischer.)

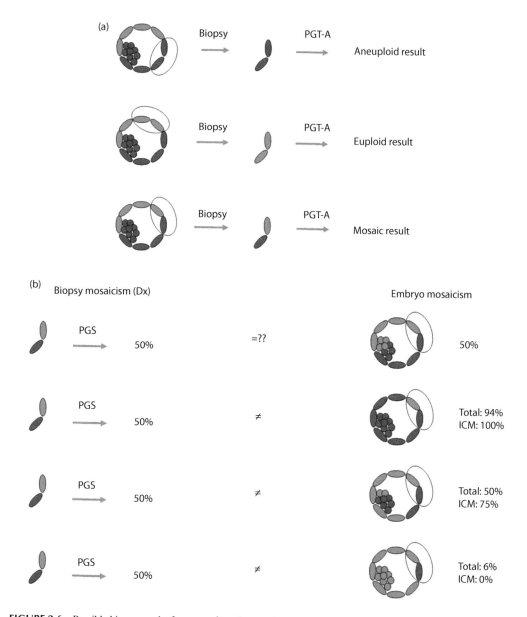

FIGURE 2.6 Possible biopsy results from mosaic embryos. (Courtesy of Alyssa Snyder, Igenomix.)

Key points for discussion regarding transfer of blastocysts with mosaic aneuploid results include:

- The clinic's storage and transfer policies for mosaic embryos (to be discussed with the patient prior to initiating a cycle).
- At the time of writing, data suggest the following, but are limited and should be interpreted with caution:
  - Lower implantation rates and higher miscarriage rates have been observed and should be expected following transfer of mosaic embryos compared to euploid embryos [27].
  - There are a small number of apparently healthy live births following conception with embryos diagnosed as mosaic [28].

- In the prenatal and pediatric populations, mosaicism involving nearly every chromosome has been reported in association with adverse outcomes. Although the magnitude of risk for adverse outcomes with pregnancies resulting from transfer of mosaic embryos is currently unknown, patients should be counseled on these risks.
- Prenatal genetic counseling and testing is strongly recommended for any pregnancy resulting from the transfer of a mosaic embryo. Testing should be offered via amniocentesis such that fetal, not placental, cells are tested. Additional analyses beyond routine karyotyping should be considered depending on the specific PGT-A result and may include:
  - Additional cell counts, in an effort to identify lower-level mosaicism
  - Chromosomal microarray, if a partial chromosome aneuploidy is involved
  - Uniparental disomy studies, depending on the chromosome involved [29]
- Postnatal evaluation by peripheral blood karyotype and/or microarray may be considered, particularly if prenatal diagnosis is declined. Referral to a pediatric genetics clinic is recommended in the event of an abnormal physical or developmental phenotype.

PGT for Monogenic Disease (PGT-M)

Techniques used for PGT for single-gene disorders have also evolved. Initial testing was performed solely by direct mutation analysis. Contamination detecting markers were added in subsequent years. The phenomenon of allele dropout came to the forefront after misdiagnoses, specifically in compound heterozygote embryos for an autosomal recessive disease. This prompted increased use of linked markers to support direct mutation analysis. Linkage could also be used when the mutation could not be tested directly solely or in conjunction with detection of the normal allele. The application of the SNP microarray analysis to embryo testing allowed for further evolution of PGT-M, utilizing linkage analysis of SNPs within, upstream, and downstream of the gene in question.

Single-gene disorder cases are the most involved cases for the genetic counselor in the IVF clinic as well as the PGT laboratory given the complex case preparation. Once referred to the PGT laboratory for PGT-M, an intake will be completed by telephone with the patient. The intake includes thorough explanation of the case preparation process and timeline, testing technique, completion of medical and family histories inclusive of a pedigree, and review of appropriate genetic testing reports on necessary family members. If any necessary reports are not available, these will be requested, and results confirmed and received prior to test creation. If necessary, for family members who have not undergone testing, the PGT laboratory genetic counselor will work with the genetic counselor at the IVF center or a genetic counselor local to the family members to arrange for such testing. Once all the required reports are received and the case is approved by the genetic counselor and molecular teams, the test creation can proceed. The PGT laboratory genetic counselor then arranges for appropriate DNA samples to be sent to the laboratory. These can be blood, saliva, buccal swabs, or extracted DNA depending on the test technique and creation process. Should DNA be available from a deceased family member or previous pregnancy, the genetic counselor arranges for it to be sent to the PGT laboratory. The PGT laboratory genetic counselor provides updates to the patient and IVF center throughout the test creation process.

Once the PGT-M test is ready, the PGT laboratory genetic counselor can conduct a follow-up consult via phone. Medical and family histories are reviewed again to include any updates. As it can be some weeks since the patient's initial consultation to the time of PGT-M setup completion, patients are reminded of the details including test technique specific to their case; benefits, risks and limitations of the test; accuracy; transfer decisions; how results will be reported; the possibility of no normal results; and follow-up testing options once pregnant. The transfer decisions discussion includes topics such as transfer of carriers and hierarchy of such if each parent has a different mutation for an autosomal recessive disorder or transfer of female carriers for X-linked recessive conditions based on chance to be symptomatic and symptoms thereof for female carriers. A letter detailing the consult is then sent to the referring IVF center physician and available to the patient.

Upon completion of testing of the embryos, results are forwarded to the IVF center. The genetic counselor at the center can review the results in detail with the patient. If the IVF center does not employ a genetic counselor, the results can be reported to the patient by the physician or clinic staff. The genetic counselor at the PGT laboratory is available to discuss the results with the IVF center or the patient directly if requested.

PGT for Structural Rearrangements (PGT-SR)

Like the test techniques for other indications for PGT, PGT-SR for chromosomal rearrangements, such as reciprocal and Robertsonian translocations and inversions, has evolved since its inception. Techniques have included breakpoint spanning probes, conversion plus FISH painting probes, polar body analysis with painting probes, subtelomeric and centromeric probes, enumerator probes for Robertsonian translocations, aCGH, and NGS. Both aCGH and NGS provide significant advancement in PGT-SR by allowing analysis of the structural aberration and aneuploidy of all other chromosomes. Currently, NGS is the method of choice for PGT-SR.

PGT-SR cases do require more scrutiny than PGT-A tests, but typically no longer require any case test preparation beyond review of parental karyotypes. The PGT laboratory genetic counselor reviews each chromosomal aberration to determine if the size of the translocated, deleted, or duplicated segments will be able to be detected by the test technique. Techniques such as aCGH and NGS detect ≥ 5 Mb and ≥ 3 Mb, respectively [23], whereas FISH is able to detect much smaller segments and may rarely still be the PGT-SR method of choice. Of note, access to such FISH-based methodology is extremely limited. For reciprocal translocations, if at least three of the translocated segments are large enough to be detected, the aCGH or NGS can be done. Best practice is to confirm a normal karyotype for the partner of a patient with a structural rearrangement.

Once accepted, the PGT laboratory genetic counselor conducts a genetic consult by phone, which includes detailed review of medical and family histories; number of segregates and percent normal/balanced; genes in the regions of breakpoints; aneuploidy, non-disjunction, and age-related statistics; details of the PGT-SR test; benefits, risks, and limitations of the test; accuracy; how results will be reported; the possibility of no normal results; and follow-up testing options once pregnant.

It is crucial to discuss the number of possible segregates and typical percent of normal/balanced embryos detected. The reciprocal translocation results in 16 possible segregates, and the Robertsonian in 6. This translates to an average of 0–2 ($\leq 20\%$) embryos detected as normal/balanced per case, not including aneuploid results. These numbers and results typically are a surprise to patients. When first diagnosed with a reciprocal translocation, most patients are counseled with the simplistic visual aid and percentages of four outcomes: one normal, one balanced, and two unbalanced. This is likely done to provide a rudimentary overview at time of diagnosis. Also, the majority of unbalanced forms do not result in a viable outcome barring a translocation with small telomeric translocated segments or some segregates of an acrocentric:non-acrocentric reciprocal translocation. Therefore, if conceiving naturally, a patient will not experience detection of all 16 segregates in their children. In contrast to this, all segregates can be detected via PGT-SR as it is the embryo being studied. Nevertheless, this change in statistic from 50% to $\leq 20\%$ per cycle being normal/balanced often induces distress and anxiety in the patient (Figures 2.7 and 2.8).

Another main concept to impart to the patient is that the current typical test detects unbalanced results but cannot differentiate balanced from normal results, as both have the same amount of chromosomal material present; these tests study quantity of material, not structure of the chromosomes. Overall, most patients accept this limitation given they themselves have a balanced form of the chromosomal rearrangement.

Like the PGT-M test results, PGT-SR test results are forwarded to the IVF center. Again, the genetic counselor or other clinician at the center will review the results in detail with the patient. The genetic counselor at the PGT laboratory is available to discuss the results with the IVF center and again will discuss results with the patient if requested by the referring center.

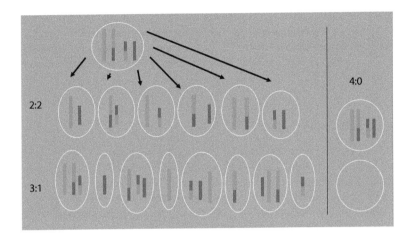

FIGURE 2.7   The 16 segregates of a reciprocal translocation. (Courtesy of Jill Fischer, Reprogenetics.)

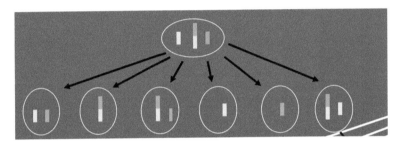

FIGURE 2.8   The six segregates of a Robertsonian translocation. (Courtesy of Jill Fischer, Reprogenetics.)

Laboratory Genetic Counseling Services

In addition to genetic counseling discussed previously, many genetics laboratories offer focused test-specific pre- and/or post-test consultations by phone to patients provided by their laboratory-based genetic counselors. Pretest consultations are an informed consent process which typically include review of the indication, test technique, and benefits, risks, and limitations of the test. A consult letter is typically generated, documenting the discussion. Laboratory genetic counselors can also review test results with patients. Overall, laboratory genetic counselors are ideal resources for patients and clinicians alike in assessing which of their laboratory's tests would be most appropriate for a specific patient. It is important to note the differences between these laboratory-based test-related genetic consultations and formal comprehensive genetic counseling. Unlike comprehensive genetic counseling discussed in this chapter, these test-specific consultations may not involve a review of the family medical history, patients' medical records, or a detailed genetic risk assessment unless it is relevant to the test being offered. Documentation of consultative services offered by laboratory genetic counselors will often note that their services are not intended to replace comprehensive genetic counseling. These test-specific services should be considered complementary to comprehensive genetic counseling services.

Additional Roles for Genetic Counselors in an ART Setting

Numerous professional societies, including ASRM, the American College of Obstetricians and Gynecologists (ACOG), and the American College of Medical Genetics and Genomics (ACMG) recommend referral of patients to a qualified genetics healthcare provider, such as a certified genetic counselor, for genetic risk assessment, testing recommendations, and management [30,31].

Beyond the immediate management of PGT details, genetic counselors in an ART setting can assist in various other activities including clinical and research protocol establishment and implementation, consent and report creation, patient follow-up and outcome data collection and presentation, and staff education.

Genetic carrier screening protocols are crucial for the ART practice. Genetic counselors are increasingly helpful in the creation and implementation of these protocols as carrier screening expands beyond testing individual genes to large multigene panels.

As patients have successful pregnancies after PGT, ART-based genetic counselors can help them navigate the various prenatal testing options in the context of the PGT that was performed in their IVF cycle. ART genetic counselors can also contribute to fluid communication and continuity of care to the obstetricians and prenatal genetic counselors who will be caring for these patients during pregnancy. Although there may be discussion of various noninvasive (screening) and invasive (diagnostic) prenatal testing options during the pre- and post PGT consultations, these details may not become fully relevant and clear for the patient until a time in their pregnancy when they are faced with such decision-making.

In the unfortunate event of a fetal anomaly or demise after PGT, the genetic counselor can facilitate appropriate testing and interpretation that may inform future treatment.

Genetic counselors can also serve as coordinators of pregnancy outcome data after PGT to ensure accurate outcome data publication for the clinic and the PGT laboratory as well as accurate reporting to organizations such as the Society for Assisted Reproductive Technologies (SART). Additionally, genetic counselors can assist in investigating any discrepancies between PGT and pre- or postnatal genetic test results.

Due to their detailed training in medical genetics and genetic technologies, genetic counselors are ideal for implementing best practices for genetic testing and overseeing clinic policy for the provision of genetic services. Putting such practices in place can help limit the clinic's liability as a result of non-genetics specialists who are less familiar with genetic testing guidelines and emerging technologies, and who are at increased risk of providing potentially inaccurate genetic information. Documentation of genetic risk assessment and testing recommendations by a certified genetic counselor can further reduce medical-legal risk.

Having a dedicated genetic counselor allows physicians, nurses, medical assistants, and embryologists to focus on delivering services specific to their areas of expertise and interest. In addition, genetic counselors are an excellent resource when it comes to ongoing genetic education for clinical staff members.

Means of Incorporating Genetic Counseling Services into an ART Clinic

There are various types of professional relationships possible for incorporating genetic counseling services into an ART clinic. Most familiar is the traditional relationship of employer/employee in which the genetic counselor is hired full- or part-time by the clinic. Other options include:

- Hiring a genetic counselor as a contract employee. Reimbursement for services rendered can be negotiated on a per diem, per patient, or per service type basis, and the genetic counselor's role in the clinic has the potential to expand as the need for genetic services increases.

- Coordinating with a local genetics clinic, such as a prenatal diagnosis center. In so doing, the same genetic counselor could see a patient both preconceptionally and prenatally.

- Contracting with a telemedicine genetic counseling service provider. These consultations may be offered by telephone or video conferencing, which can be convenient for the patient, especially if they are not geographically close to the IVF center. Unlike the IVF clinic-based genetic counselor, telemedicine genetic counseling services are typically purely consultative, and the arrangement, ordering, and management of any recommended genetic testing falls to the referring provider. However, a telemedicine genetic counseling service can aid with accurate interpretation of any genetic test results.

With each of these modalities, it is typical for the genetic counselor to provide the physician and patient with a written genetic counseling summary report.

How Can I Find a Genetic Counselor?

The NSGC (www.nsgc.org) and ABGC (www.abgc.net) websites offer a "find a genetic counselor" search function that allows searching by region, specialty, and/or name. These websites also offer job posting services through e-mail blasts to their membership to assist potential employers in finding qualified genetic counselors to incorporate into their clinical practices.

REFERENCES

1. National Society of Genetic Counselors (NSGC). Available from www.nsgc.org. Accessed on March 7, 2020.
2. The 2018 Jobs Rated Report. Available from https://www.careercast.com/jobs-rated/2018-jobs-rated-report. Accessed March 7, 2020.
3. Snider S. 25 Amazing Health Care Support Jobs for 2017. *U.S. News and World Report.* Available from https://money.usnews.com/careers/slideshows/25-amazing-health-care-support-jobs-for-2017?slide=13. 2017 and updated 2019. Accessed March 7, 2020.
4. *U.S. News and World Report* Best Jobs Rankings. Best Health Care Support Jobs. Available from https://money.usnews.com/careers/best-jobs/rankings/best-health-care-support-jobs. 2018. Accessed March 7, 2020.
5. Bureau of Labor Statistics, U.S. Department of Labor. *Occupational Outlook Handbook*, Genetic Counselors. Available from https://www.bls.gov/ooh/healthcare/genetic-counselors.htm. Accessed March 7, 2020.
6. Supreme Court of the United States. Syllabus Association for Molecular Pathology et. al. v. Myriad Genetic Inc. et. el. Available from https://www.supremecourt.gov/opinions/12pdf/12-398_1b7d.pdf. 2013. Accessed March 7, 2020.
7. Barnes R, Dennis B. Supreme Court rules human genes may not be patented. *The Washington Post.* Available from https://www.washingtonpost.com/politics/supreme-court-rules-human-genes-may-not-be-patented/2013/06/13/9e5c55d2-d43d-11e2-a73e-826d299ff459_story.html?noredirect=on&utm_term=.52add24af940. 2013. Accessed March 7, 2020.
8. Bookman T. Kaiser Health News. A shortage of genetic counselors. *The Atlantic.* Available from https://www.theatlantic.com/health/archive/2016/04/shortage-of-genetic-counselors/478815/. 2016. Accessed March 7, 2020.
9. Association Council for Genetic Counseling (ACGC). Accreditation Manual for Master's Degree Genetic Counseling Programs. Available from https://www.gceducation.org/standards-of-accreditation/ Accessed March 7, 2020.
10. Association Council for Genetic Counseling (ACGC). Accredited Programs. Available from http://gceducation.org/Pages/Accredited-Programs.aspx. Accessed March 7, 2020.
11. Ormond KE et al. Genetic Counseling Globally: Where are we now? *Am J Med Genet.* 2018;178(1):98–107.
12. Do I Qualify? Available from https://www.abgc.net/becoming-certified/do-i-qualify/. Accessed March 7, 2020.
13. Why Get Certified? Available from https://www.abgc.net/becoming-certified/why-get-certified/. Accessed March 7, 2020.
14. California Department of Public Health Genetic Counselor Licensure Program. Genetic Counselor Title Protection Information. Available from https://www.cdph.ca.gov/Programs/CFH/DGDS/Pages/psqa/Frequently%20Asked%20Questions%20Pages/Genetic-Counselor-Title-Protection.aspx. Accessed March 7, 2020.
15. Certification Process. Available from https://www.abgc.net/becoming-certified/certification-process/. Accessed March 7, 2020.
16. States Issuing Licenses for Genetic Counselors. Available from https://www.nsgc.org/p/cm/ld/fid=19. Accessed March 7, 2020.
17. Uhlmann WR et al. *A Guide to Genetic Counseling.* 2nd Ed. Wiley-Blackwell; 2009;ISBN-13: 978-0470179659.

18. Who Are Genetic Counselors? Available from https://www.nsgc.org/page/whoaregcs. Accessed March 7, 2020.

19. Weil J. Psychosocial genetic counseling in the post-nondirective era: A point of view. *J Genet Couns.* 2003;12(3):199–211.

20. Ethics Committee of ASRM. Transferring embryos with genetic anomalies detected in preimplantation testing: an Ethics Committee opinion. *Fertil Steril.* 2017;107:1130–5.

21. DeRycke M et al. ESHRE PGD Consortium data collection XIV-XV: Cycles from January 2011 to December 2012 with pregnancy follow up to October 2013. *Hum Reprod.* 2017;32(10):1974–94.

22. Practice Committees of ASRM and SART. The use of preimplantation genetic testing for aneuploidy (PGT-A): A committee opinion. *Fertil Steril.* 2018;109:429–36.

23. Munné S. Preimplantation genetic diagnosis for aneuploidy and translocations using array comparative genomic hybridization. *Curr Genomics.* 2012;13(6):463–70.

24. Munné S, Wells, D. Detection of mosaicism at the blastocyst stage with the use of high-resolution next-generation sequencing. *Fertil Steril.* 2017;107(5):1085–91.

25. Preimplantation Genetic Diagnosis International Society. PGDIS position statement on chromosome mosaicism and preimplantation aneuploidy testing at the blastocyst stage. *PGDIS Newsletter.* July 19, 2016. Available at: http://www.pgdis.org/docs/newsletter_071816.html. Accessed June 9, 2018.

26. CoGEN. CoGEN Position Statement on Chromosomal Mosaicism Detected in Preimplantation Blastocyst Biopsies. 2016. https://ivf-worldwide.com/cogen/general/cogen-statement.html. Accessed July 3, 2018.

27. Fragouli E et al. Analysis of implantation and ongoing pregnancy rates following the transfer of mosaic diploid–aneuploid blastocysts. *Hum Genet.* 2017;136:805.

28. Greco E, Minasi MG, Fiorentino F. Healthy babies after intrauterine transfer of mosaic aneuploid blastocysts. *N Engl J Med.* 2015;373:2089–90.

29. Shaffer L, Agan N, Goldberg J, Ledbetter D, Longshore J, Cassidy S. American College of Medical Genetics Statement on Diagnostic Testing for Uniparental Disomy. *Genet Med.* 2001;3(3):206–11.

30. The Practice Committee of ASRM and SART. Recommendations for gamete and embryo donation: a committee opinion. *Fertil Steril.* 2013;99:47–62.

31. Edwards JG et al. Expanded carrier screening in reproductive medicine-points to consider: A Joint Statement of the American College of Medical Genetics and Genomics, American College of Obstetricians and Gynecologists, National Society of Genetic Counselors, Perinatal Quality Foundation, and Society for Maternal-Fetal Medicine. *Obstet Gynecol.* 2015;125(3):653–62.

3

Preimplantation Genetic Testing for Aneuploidies: Where We Are and Where We're Going

Andrea Victor, Cagri Ogur, Alan Thornhill, and Darren K. Griffin

CONTENTS

Introduction

The most prominent and controversial use for preimplantation genetic testing (PGT) is for aneuploidy testing of oocytes and embryos (PGT-A). PGT-A serves a threefold purpose. First, it tests for chromosomal aneuploidies that can lead to the birth of babies with chromosomal copy number syndromes (e.g., Down syndrome—trisomy 21). Second, it has the potential to reduce miscarriage rates, as approximately half of all first trimester abortions are chromosomally abnormal. Finally, it is often prescribed with the intention of improving *in vitro* fertilization (IVF) outcomes, e.g., by reducing time to pregnancy.

Brief History

PGT technology was first applied to rabbits in the late 1960s, detecting the presence of Barr bodies—inactive sex chromosomes (their presence being indicative of female sex), thereby chronicling the first example of PGT [1]. The first reported use of PGT in humans, however, involved polymerase chain reaction (PCR) of Y-specific repeat sequences in order to detect the presence of the Y chromosome and hence also determine sex. By only transferring female embryos, the transmission of X-linked conditions in which the mother was a carrier [2] could be controlled, such that none of the progeny would be affected. The detection of a Y-specific sequence was, however, extremely prone to both false positive and false negative results and was soon replaced by fluorescence *in-situ* hybridization (FISH) technology [3,4], detecting X-and Y-specific probes in a dual color strategy.

Cytogenetic detection of sex chromosomes preceded the idea of testing embryos for chromosomal aneuploidies. At its inception, the goal of PGT-A was to reduce the risk of offspring with live-born chromosomal syndromes. FISH technology was used to obtain copy number information of high-risk chromosomes 13, 18, 21, X, and Y [5,6]. Embryos that did not have the normal complement of targeted chromosomes could then be deselected for transfer.

The panel of screened chromosomes soon grew to include chromosomes 16 and 22, both of which are common in spontaneous abortions [7]. Notably, screening of chromosomal abnormalities associated with increased miscarriage prior to implantation marked a seminal shift in the previously limited uses of PGT. Such studies signified the first instances of harnessing this technology beyond reducing the risk of disease in offspring and broadened its application to improving IVF outcomes. As such, exploiting this technology in this manner facilitated achieving viable pregnancies more likely to result in healthy live births while reducing the risk of miscarriage. Referral categories, therefore, included treatment of patients experiencing recurrent miscarriage (RM) and recurrent implantation failure (RIF) [8]. Additionally, cited uses include the treatment of patients of advanced maternal age (AMA) [8] —the most common use of PGT-A—and severe male factor infertility [9,10], both of which result in increased levels of embryonic aneuploidy.

Although 24-chromosome FISH was eventually reported [11,12], technical limitations prevented FISH from expanding its screening panel much beyond 12 chromosomes for routine use, establishing a detection ceiling of 60%–80% of all aneuploid embryos [13]. Given that aneuploidy can affect all 24 chromosomes in the early human embryo [14], this could be a contributing factor as to why randomized controlled trials failed to show improvements in live-birth rates utilizing this technology [15,16]. Other reasons might be sub-optimal (cleavage-stage) biopsy protocols that led to embryo damage. A more comprehensive PGT-A test was thus needed if PGT-A were to be taken seriously as a means of improving IVF outcomes. Genome-wide molecular methodologies like quantitative PCR, array comparative genomic hybridization (aCGH), and next-generation sequencing (NGS) were thus introduced.

Twenty-four-chromosome screening methodologies brought with them increased resolution, offering information on the karyotype of an embryo beyond uniform whole-chromosome aneuploidy. This included the possibility of gaining insight into embryonic mosaicism and segmental aneuploidies. Such in-depth information offers practitioners and patients additional ways to select chromosomally normal embryo(s) for transfer within a cohort. Concurrently, continued advancement in the IVF laboratory has meant improved fertilization, better embryo culture systems, less damaging biopsy protocols, and higher quality embryos. In addition, improved implantation rates and refinements in cryopreservation methods have made the transfer of fewer embryos (preferably a single embryo) a categorical requirement to prevent high-risk multiple pregnancy. Taken together, these technological advancements further underscore the need for more refined, objective embryo selection methods such as those provided by PGT-A.

Looking Forward

Over the past three decades, PGT-M has been credited with the birth of thousands of unaffected children [17,18]. The efficacy of PGT-A, on the other hand, despite also boasting thousands of healthy live births from IVF cycles utilizing this technology, is still widely debated. The more abstract but pivotal application of PGT-A is not to prevent disease by inheritance, but to maximize implantation potential while addressing patients' specific needs. These individualized concerns may include a patient's anxiety over the prospect of experiencing another miscarriage or offering a young couple the peace of mind of having genetically competent embryos banked for future use. Unfortunately, while critical to good patient care, these benefits are harder to quantify and often overlooked.

According to the European Society of Human Reproduction and Embryology (ESHRE) PGD consortium data for the 10-year period of 1997–2007, out of more than 27,000 cycles that reached oocyte retrieval, over 60% were destined for aneuploidy screening. Global figures are becoming more difficult to collate but it has been estimated that approximately 100,000 PGT cycles have been performed worldwide over the past 23 years (www.pgdis.org) and nearly 80% of these cycles have been PGT-A (personal communication from numerous meetings including the PGD International Society [PGDIS]). The demand of IVF has been increasing due to wider accessibility and various societal trends, and with it, so it seems, the use of PGT-A. Nonetheless, the efficacy of PGT-A and its clinical applicability continues to be questioned and debated. Numerous studies attest to its efficacy including retrospective analyses, randomized controlled trials, and non-selection studies. However, the majority of these have attracted criticism either for sample size, study design, or interpretation. Most recently, a large multicenter trial (the STAR trial) [19] provided ammunition for both proponents and opponents of PGT-A. For the latter, analysis suggested no significant increase in improving first-time pregnancy rates overall. Reanalysis of the data, however, for women over the age of 35 demonstrated a significant improvement. Moreover, the study provided clear evidence that procedural or technical differences between IVF centers can influence PGT-A outcomes.

The Impact of Sampling Methods on PGT-A and the Advantages of Vitrification

In keeping with all forms of PGT, there are three sources from which cells can be biopsied for use in PGT-A. These are polar bodies from oocytes, blastomeres from cleavage-stage embryos, and trophectoderm cells from blastocysts. In an ideal world, the timing of biopsy should be to ensure the most accurate identification of chromosome imbalance, and the result on the biopsied cell(s) should correlate to an identical abnormality in the remainder of the embryo. Biopsy timing also affects the decision of whether to vitrify all of the embryos ("freeze all") or perform embryo transfer using fresh embryos in the first cycle.

Polar Body Biopsy

Polar body (PB) biopsy was first introduced to identify oocytes that carry disease alleles in women heterozygous for a genetic disease [20]. Polar bodies are the byproducts of meiosis I and II, and their biopsy is not likely to impact negatively on an embryo's future development. Polar bodies may be removed either one at a time or simultaneously following fertilization [21], but because they might undergo rapid fragmentation, any delay in biopsy could result in misdiagnosis or no result. The primary advantages of polar body biopsy are that it is less invasive than other forms and it inherently creates a greater time window for analysis when performing transfer for a fresh cycle. Disadvantages lie in the fact that polar bodies cannot be used to detect paternal chromosomes or post-zygotic errors. Consequently, polar body biopsy is limited in PGT-A to the diagnosis of meiotic abnormalities and translocations of maternal origin. Polar body biopsy gained popularity when it was proposed as an alternative to cleavage-stage biopsy [22,23], which, after randomized controlled trials (RCTs) [15,24], limited the applicability of PGT-A. Indeed, the first successful live birth following 24-chromosome screening was performed following polar body biopsy [25].

Detecting chromosome segregation errors following polar body biopsy is limited to meiotic abnormalities. This is an important limitation because analysis on serial biopsies of embryos has demonstrated that approximately half the embryos (47.6%) found to have an abnormality carry aneuploidies other than female meiotic-derived ones [26]. Indeed, analysis of polar body biopsy material has the least predictive value for whole embryo ploidy and implantation potential compared to the other two methods [27]. Moreover, prediction of the ploidy status of PBs with reciprocal aneuploidies (e.g., where the first polar body has disomy 21 and the second has nullisomy 21) raises another issue: that is, reciprocal aneuploidies of the same chromosomes are nearly always from a euploid embryo [28]. A further consideration is the differentiation between single chromatid and whole chromosome losses and gains, when single chromosome losses are the most prevalent. It has been suggested that pooling first and second polar body ahead of DNA amplification could alleviate this problem and reduce costs [29].

A recent multicenter RCT involving 23-chromosome testing of polar bodies for PGT-A (using the array CGH platform—see as follows) was performed (the ESHRE Study Into The Evaluation of Oocyte Euploidy by Microarray Analysis [ESTEEM]) [30] involving women aged 36–41. Primary results were deemed "disappointing" because the likelihood of a live birth within 1 year did not increase. One positive result, however, was that the miscarriage rate was significantly lower than the "no intervention" group [31], which may provide a sufficient incentive for some patients.

Cleavage-Stage (Blastomere) Biopsy

Blastomere (cleavage-stage) biopsy is performed by the removal of one or two cells from a day 3 embryo that has at least six cells. Calcium (Ca^{2+}) and Magnesium (Mg^{2+})-free media is commonly used to reverse compaction facilitating cell removal. In order to open the zona pellucida chemical (acid Tyrode's solution), mechanical or, most commonly, laser-assisted, approaches may be used. This approach assesses both maternal and paternal contributions to the embryo and allows sufficient time for analysis to be performed before transfer of a fresh embryo, even if transport PGT (i.e., sending samples to specialist diagnostic labs) is used. This technique is the oldest and, until recently, the most widely applied method for PGT-A [17] but nonetheless is prone to technical and biological drawbacks. First, the mosaicism rate is at its highest level in cleavage-stage embryos, regardless of maternal age; moreover, the potential damage of a significantly decreasing cell number on further development is significant [32].

Cleavage-stage biopsy was probably behind the biggest controversies surrounding PGT-A. Some initial retrospective studies proved positive [6,33], but later RCTs demonstrated either no improvement or an adverse effect on IVF outcome [15,34]. The subsequent melee that ensued shows little sign of abating, with some arguing PGT-A in its entirety should be discontinued on the basis of these results, but others making the point that it is cleavage-stage biopsy that is the problem. With a mean of eight cells, removing one or two incurs the serious risk of impeding an embryo's developmental potential, and could be operator dependent. The initial RCTs were in fact severely criticized on the basis that one interpretation of the Mastenbroek et al. [15] data is that there was a third group in the manuscript (briefly mentioned) that had biopsy but no PGT-A. A 6% live-birth rate in this group compared to 16.8% in the PGT-A cohort (and 14.7% in controls) provides evidence, some argue, that cleavage-stage biopsy in the hands of these particular authors may be the root cause of these adverse outcomes.

The effect of cleavage-stage biopsy on developing embryos was assessed in an RCT using a paired design [35]. That study demonstrated a relative 39% reduction in implantation rates as a result of cleavage-stage biopsy but no measurable adverse effect after trophectoderm biopsy [35]. There is also some evidence from morphokinetic analysis that developmental dynamics are impaired after blastomere biopsy, causing delayed compaction and altered hatching [36,37]. A further drawback of blastomere biopsy is that with only one cell to analyze and the relatively high mosaicism rate, the process is prone to false positive and negative results. Taking all these things into account, cleavage-stage biopsy has largely been discontinued and replaced by blastocyst-stage (trophectoderm) biopsy for all forms of PGT.

Blastocyst-Stage (Trophectoderm) Biopsy

Blastocyst-stage (trophectoderm) biopsy became the most commonly used PGT-A method after improved culture conditions have led to much higher blastulation rates [38]. Trophectoderm biopsy can either be performed directly on a day 5–7 blastocyst or by the biopsy of a small part of the trophectoderm herniates through the opening previously created on day 3.

Trophectoderm biopsy has many advantages. First, the blastocyst has >100 cells, and thus the removal of between two and ten cells is less likely to have an adverse effect on future embryo development. As a result of having more cells to analyze, amplification failure, misdiagnosis, and allele dropout (ADO) are lower compared to cleavage-stage biopsy [39] and there is evidence that mosaicism is lower in blastocysts compared to cleavage-stage IVF embryos [40]. Using this natural selective advantage, the cytogenetic analysis of blastocysts not only reduces the relative cost of PGT-A, but also reportedly increases implantation rate and multiple pregnancy risk as a result of single euploid blastocyst transfer [41,42]. Moreover, there has been a suggestion that the trophectoderm biopsy technique is possibly less operator dependent and thus more reproducible across various IVF clinics [43]. For this reason, RCTs demonstrating benefits of PGT-A were carried out using trophectoderm [19,41,44,45] except for one that used cleavage-stage biopsy [46], which also demonstrated the benefits of PGT-A.

The Impact of Vitrification and "Freeze-All" Strategies

In fresh cycles, the time for analysis is limited by the implantation window of the blastocyst. Cryopreservation is thus an attractive option, at least for subsequent cycles, and this was initially thought to be a major drawback. Despite this, the development of enhanced culture conditions and improved vitrification techniques led to improved blastulation rates, more embryos available for trophectoderm biopsy, and improved survival post-thawing [47]. Indeed, IVF (regardless of PGT) has seen improvement in embryo cryopreservation techniques, and recently there has been a change in emphasis toward embryo vitrification with a view to a deferred transfer ("freeze-all") to reduce or eliminate the possibility of ovarian hyperstimulation syndrome. Therefore, while to some degree increased pregnancy success rates have been associated with PGT-A technologies getting better (i.e., improved blastocyst biopsy and 24-chromosome screening), improved vitrification and "freeze-all" may play a part. The transfer of previously vitrified single blastocysts reportedly leads to equivalent live-birth rates and improved neonatal outcomes compared to fresh transfers [48]. An additional factor is the improved knowledge of the endometrium in determining the window of implantation through studies of the endometrial transcriptome [49,50]. In frozen embryo transfer cycles, natural or modified natural regimes appear to be superior to conventional medicated regimes, when gene expression profiles are used to determine implantation window [51]. Moreover, transfer in subsequent cycles may also allow for preparation of a more physiological and receptive endometrium, e.g., through consideration of the microbiome.

Technical Issues with Chromosome Analysis

Depending on the developmental stage at which the biopsy is performed, between one and ten cells (but typically no more than five from a blastocyst) are removed from the embryo and used for testing. Like most diagnostic tests, a high level of accuracy is required given the potential ramifications of a misdiagnosis. A false negative result would mean an abnormal embryo is diagnosed as normal and could result in miscarriage, ongoing pregnancy, or live birth of a chromosomally abnormal baby. Alternatively, a false positive may result in a chromosomally normal embryo being misdiagnosed and discarded.

Fluorescence *In-Situ* Hybridization

FISH utilizes fluorescently labeled DNA sequences (probes) to visualize specific chromosomal regions. The probes contain complementary sequences that bind to a region of interest and can be visualized using fluorescent microscopy. When applied in the context of PGT-A, biopsied cell(s) from gametes/ embryos are fixed to a slide. Probes are hybridized to the fixed material, and the presence or absence of each targeted chromosomal region is indicated by whether or not the fluorescent tags/signals are present under a fluorescent microscope. It is inferred that the presence of a signal indicates the chromosome is present, while its absence indicates it is missing.

Though the technique was developed in the 1980s, its first use in the IVF clinic was not until 1992, when it was used as an alternative to PCR-based methods to treat families at risk of transmitting sex-linked disorders by probing for chromosome X and Y [4,52]. Shortly thereafter, FISH was applied to assess the chromosomal copy number of an embryo, by probing for chromosomes associated with live-born syndromes (13, 18, 21, X, and Y), thereby establishing the first iteration of PGT-A. Over time, FISH panels used for PGT-A increased to include up to 12 chromosomes, starting with those known to display the highest frequency of aneuploidy in material from first-trimester spontaneous abortion and prenatal loss. Later additions included chromosomes associated with high levels of aneuploidy in the early developing embryo [53].

The number of chromosomes that could be targeted, however, was limited by the spectral resolution, filter sets, and the small amount of embryonic material available for testing. That is, although 24-chromosome FISH was eventually achieved [11,12], this was more applicable as a research tool and never likely to be applied clinically. While 5- to 12-chromosome panel FISH was a widespread diagnostic technology in the IVF labs of the 1990s, as a clinically reliable diagnostic tool, it has substantial limitations and challenges. As only a single target on each chromosome is probed, any segmental abnormality outside of this region would go undiagnosed, underscoring the limited resolution of the test. In addition, cell nucleus fixation and downstream analysis are technically challenging, operator dependent, and subjective. Finally, probe failures and overlapping signals are not uncommon and can significantly hinder an accurate diagnosis in an already limited chromosomal panel. These drawbacks are likely to be some of the principal reasons why RCTs have failed to show improved live-birth rates in PGT-A IVF cycles using this technology [15,16].

FISH is still occasionally used for chromosomal screening of human embryos in certain clinics, but it has largely been replaced by genome-wide molecular techniques. Though it continues to be used in instances of inherited structural rearrangements where breakpoints cannot be adequately diagnosed using PCR-based methods (see PGT-SR in Chapter 4), it is mostly relegated to research practices in IVF and PGT in the investigation of nuclear organization and mosaicism [54].

The Need for Whole-Genome Amplification to Facilitate 24-Chromosome Screening

A major limitation of preimplantation genetic testing is the limited amount of starting material—polar bodies from a mature oocyte or zygote, one or two blastomeres from a cleavage-stage embryo, or five (to ten) cells from a blastocyst. With each cell containing approximately 6 pg of DNA, even a ten-cell biopsy does not yield sufficient DNA to meet the current required input quantities for molecular testing approaches like aCGH and NGS. To meet the needs of higher-resolution molecular techniques, new technology was called for.

Whole-genome amplification (WGA) methods were developed in the early 1990s as a means to increase the amount of DNA from limited samples in a sequence-independent fashion. It quickly became an invaluable tool in the world of molecular genetics, as it made copy number variation in single or few cell samples possible. The field of embryo testing welcomed the technology, as it addressed the issue of insufficient sample size.

There are various types of WGA, which fall broadly into three categories: PCR based, multiple displacement amplification (MDA) based, and hybrid. Each approach has advantages and disadvantages when it comes to important features like genome coverage, representation bias, reproducibility, error rates, robustness, and yield. PCR-based methods include degenerate oligonucleotide-primed PCR (DOP-PCR), which utilizes partially degenerate oligonucleotide sequences/primers, thermostable DNA polymerase, and slowly increasing annealing temperatures during the PCR reaction. It is a relatively short two-step protocol that can be completed in less than 3 hours [55]. Recent modifications in the reaction chemistry have significantly improved the quality of the amplified material by providing increased genome coverage and decreased allele dropout (ADO) [56]. DOPlify, a popular commercial DOP-PCR kit, has been integrated into various downstream genome-wide PGT-A workflows.

Also loosely falling into the PCR-based WGA category are linker-adapter PCR (LA-PCR) methodologies. In LA-PCR, template DNA is fragmented and tagmented, meaning linkers containing a primer binding site are enzymatically attached to the ends of the fragmented DNA. PCR is then used to amplify the tagmented DNA fragments by adding PCR primers complementary to the linker-primer binder site. While this method can be more labor intensive than other amplification methods, it appears to offer reasonable reproducibility and genome uniformity, allowing for accurate chromosome copy number assessment. This is leveraged in various downstream genome-wide workflows, as various commercially available LA-PCR kits, like Sureplex and Picoplex, are currently some of the most widely used WGA chemistries for PGT-A purposes.

MDA is a non-PCR-based method for WGA. MDA uses high-fidelity bacteriophage DNA polymerase that denatures double-stranded DNA and amplifies a single-stranded template in an isothermal reaction. The high-fidelity polymerase reduces nucleotide errors in amplified sequences, which is well suited for single nucleotide polymorphism (SNP) detection; however, its amplification uniformity across the genome appears hampered compared to PCR-based methods [57]. Though minimal hands-on time is required, the reaction time can be greater than 8 hours.

Hybrid WGA techniques combine MDA and LA-PCR methodologies, like multiple annealing and looping-based amplification cycles (MALBAC). An initial isothermal amplification of denatured template is performed using specific MALBAC primers, followed by PCR amplification of the DNA-MALBAC primer fragments. Hybrid methods, though more labor intensive than standard MDA, offer reasonable uniformity across the genome [57–60].

WGA chemistries and the availability of more DNA from PGT samples ushered in a new era of molecular diagnostic techniques requiring starting material beyond just a few cells.

Comparative Genomic Hybridization

Comparative genomic hybridization (CGH) is a method for analyzing copy number variations (CNVs) of a sample by comparing it to the ploidy status of a reference sample. Applying the principles of FISH, the process of CGH also utilizes DNA hybridization. However, instead of hybridizing labeled probes to a fixed sample, CGH involves fluorescently labeling sample DNA (in red) and a known euploid reference DNA (in green). These samples are then cohybridized to a normal metaphase spread to bind to their locus of origin. With the help of a fluorescent microscope and software, the differentially colored fluorescent signals are compared along the length of each chromosome for identification of chromosomal differences between the sample and reference. If the sample is euploid, the ratio of sample to reference DNA will be balanced and an equal mix of red and green will be seen across all chromosomes. Any chromosomal imbalance will be detected as a shift toward red or green for that specific chromosome.

CGH was first introduced as a diagnostic tool to test for chromosome copy number changes in solid tumors in the early 1990s [61]. The technology was successfully applied to the field of IVF and PGT-A in 1999, using whole-genome amplified material from single cells biopsied from cleavage-stage embryos. Unlike limited-panel FISH, CGH offered ploidy information across all 24 chromosomes [62,63]. In fact, it offered information on copy number at various loci across all 24 chromosomes and for the first time shed light on the incidence of segmental aneuploidies and genomic instabilities in preimplantation development [64].

While a breakthrough technology, this procedure was laborious and time-consuming [65]. In a clinical setting this presented challenges given the time constraints of embryo development, uterine receptivity, and window of implantation. Therefore, in order to be effectively applied in an IVF setting, CGH required embryos to be frozen and used in a future frozen embryo transfer cycle. Despite the advancements in PGT, the process of embryo freezing was not yet sufficiently advanced to support this process.

Nevertheless, this comprehensive approach provided a springboard to the development of additional genome-wide PGT-A technologies, including workflows that were more compatible with IVF cycle timing and platforms with further increased resolution, due to the new appreciation for segmental abnormalities in IVF embryos [66,67].

Array-CGH

Array CGH (aCGH) is similar to CGH in that it involves the fluorescent labeling of a sample to a known reference and assessment of copy number by comparative analysis [68]. Instead of being hybridized to metaphase chromosomes, however, the two-colored DNA sample/reference cocktail is hybridized to bacterial artificial chromosomes (BAC) or synthetic oligonucleotides, bound to glass slides in microarray format. Fluorescence ratios at each arrayed DNA element are analyzed and can provide a locus-by-locus measure of DNA copy number variation at an increased mapping resolution to standard CGH.

A fully automated aCGH solution (24Sure; BlueGnome Ltd., later acquired by Illumina, Inc.) was introduced in 2009 with a workflow that was IVF cycle–friendly and allowed for fresh embryo transfer even when biopsying advanced blastocysts. The specialized software (BlueFuse) analyzed the ratio of the fluorescent signal intensity at each chromosomal position, or clone, represented on the array, and compared these ratios to those of reference DNA. Clones with normalized intensities significantly greater than the reference intensities indicated copy number gain in the sample at that position. Similarly, significantly lower intensities in the sample are signs of copy number loss. BlueFuse software (Illumina, Inc.) calculates standard deviation ratios after smoothing and normalizing raw data [25,69–71], reporting genome-wide copy number information as log2 ratios. It is able to offer a mapping resolution as small as 2.5 Mb [72].

aCGH technology as a tool for PGT-A has been rigorously and successfully applied in the field, including proof of principle [23], preclinical validation [73], RCT [44], and retrospective case control studies [74]. Despite its numerous strengths, aCGH does have its limitations. It cannot detect polyploidies or uniparental disomies (UPD) because the relative ratios of chromosomal DNA are the same as those of the control DNA. Another disadvantage is resolution and the limited ability to detect mosaicism [75].

Next-Generation Sequencing

Sequencing is the process of determining the order of nucleotides. The "next-generation" designation refers to the more recently developed technologies that have the ability to generate this information quickly, accurately, and in a cost-effective manner. These methods started emerging in the early 2000s and catapulted the fields of biological research and medical genetics into a new era. They offer a major progression toward a more comprehensive characterization of the human genome and associated genetic disease. The field of PGT-A began harnessing these tools for routine use a decade later [76–78]. The most popular sequencing platforms utilized for PGT-A purposes include Illumina and Ion Torrent technologies. Both systems essentially entail single-stranded DNA template being repeatedly exposed to a sequence of dNTPs. Incorporation of bases complementary to the template can be detected in different ways. Illumina sequencing by synthesis technology enriches DNA templates with fluorescently labeled chain-terminating nucleotides, and base incorporation/calling is determined by light detection using specialized cameras. Ion Torrent/LifeTech technology, rather than utilizing optical components, detects nucleotide sequences by changes in pH, as nucleotide incorporation releases protons, changing the pH of the surrounding solution proportional to the number of incorporated nucleotides.

There are two basic approaches of these sequencing methodologies when applied for PGT-A analysis. One, a non-targeted, shotgun sequencing of random fragmented genomic DNA from WGA-biopsied embryonic material. And two, a targeted sequencing approach, which performs a highly multiplexed PCR to amplify many targeted regions across the genome.

Regardless of the approach, a barcoding step allows all fragments of a specific sample to have a unique identification sequence attached, or molecular barcode [79]. The ability to label each sample with a molecular signature allows multiple samples to be processed at once, providing time- and cost-saving benefits. Resulting data are demultiplexed, and individual samples are mapped to a known human reference genome. The number of reads at each chromosomal region can be quantified, and any potential aneuploidy can be deduced by a disproportionate number of reads in a given region.

PGT-A with NGS has shown increased resolution for small CNVs, structural rearrangements, and mosaicism as compared to aCGH. Moreover, NGS has the ability to simultaneously detect monogenic disorders [80]. Mosaicism detection of various NGS PGT-A workflows has been thoroughly explored, and limits of detection have been reported to be as low as 10% [81,82]. This topic is further addressed in a number of number of later sections. NGS has also increased the confidence in the detection of some polyploidy, as compared to previous technologies, although commonly used PGT-A platforms are still not able to identify this condition in all cases.

Because of these improvements, it has been suggested that NGS technology has had a positive impact on IVF outcomes by decreasing failed implantation and miscarriage rates [83].

Real-Time Quantitative PCR

Real-time quantitative PCR (qPCR) applies the same tenets as classical PCR but has the ability to offer quantitative information of PCR-targeted loci. It monitors DNA amplification as the reaction progresses by using fluorescently labeled primers such that a fluorescent signal can be recorded at each PCR cycle. Signals can be measured, and relative target abundance can be determined between template DNA and a calibrator reference sample.

Methods applying this technology to PGT-A have been described and successfully utilized in the clinic on blastocyst biopsies from advanced-stage embryos [45,85,86]. The procedure is cost effective and efficient as compared to other genome-wide PGT-A solutions and does not require the use of WGA [87,88], likely reducing the risk of amplification bias. This process involves a multiplexed preamplification reaction targeting specific loci across the genome, followed by qPCR using TaqMan copy number assay. Importantly, this method can be easily combined with testing for monogenic mutations.

One drawback, however, is its limited resolution, as it only provides copy number information at a limited number of defined regions on each chromosome. This greatly reduces its ability to detect segmental abnormalities when compared to other methodologies and could thus underreport abnormalities, leading to increased risk of miscarriage. The ability of this method to detect mosaicism, however, remains to be determined.

Single-Nucleotide Polymorphism Arrays

A single-nucleotide polymorphism (SNP) is a variation at a single site in the genome and is the most frequent type of variation found in humans. A SNP array is a technology used to detect these polymorphisms, using the same basic principles of standard microarray, including DNA hybridization, fluorescent microscopy, and solid surface capture in order to detect these polymorphisms. Unlike classic microarrays that can only detect gains or losses at a probed region, SNP arrays contain two hybridization loci per SNP. Each allele is differentially labeled, allowing for the detection of hetero- and homozygosity [89], as well as instances of allelic imbalance [90], including loss of heterozygosity (LOH) and UPD.

Though most commonly used for genome-wide association studies (GWAS) to map disease loci, SNP arrays can also be utilized to generate a virtual karyotype by using software to determine the copy number of each SNP present on the array by comparative fluorescence and subsequent alignment of the SNPs in chromosomal order. SNP technology has been successfully applied as a chromosome copy number tool in the context of PGT-A [91–93]. Benefits include comprehensive detection of polyploidy, UPD, and simultaneous detection of PGT-A and M.

Karyomapping and Haplarthymisis

Karyomapping is a high-density SNP genotyping platform that uses parental DNA to determine "informative" loci of a parental haplotype, where four distinct sets of markers can be identified across each parental chromosome [94]. Parental genotypes can be aligned with genotypes of their children and/ or embryo genotypes, generating a "karyomap" that can display homologous chromosomes and any points of genetic exchange induced by chiasmata. As such, in the event of a chromosomal abnormality, it can infer whether the abnormality has stemmed from meiosis I, meiosis II, or a post-zygotic error [95,96]. Haplarhythmisis works on a similar principle to karyomapping but also has an element of quantification [96]. The disadvantage of these approaches for aneuploidy detection is that they are limited in their ability to detect mosaicism originating from mitotic errors (see next section).

In the event of a mosaic result, the source of the chromosomal error may have substantial clinical implications. For example, it is known that meiotically incurred mosaic trisomies later corrected by trisomy rescue lead to poorer clinical outcomes as compared to mosaicism resulting from post-zygotic errors [97]. Like SNP arrays, karyomapping is also able to detect polyploidy, detect UPD, and simultaneously perform PGT-A and PGT-M testing. Due to its high cost, however, it is mainly reserved for when screening for a monogenic disorder is required.

FISH, aCGH, NGS, and SNP technologies have all been instrumental tools as we try to better understand the basic patterns of chromosome abnormalities in early human embryonic development. These insights may offer clinicians and patients decision-making tools for optimal clinical outcomes.

Aneuploidy and Mosaicism—What We Know

Aneuploidy

Aneuploidy is a disorder of chromosome number. Its classical definition in humans describes any deviation of 23 or its multiples in chromosome count. The most commonly encountered forms of aneuploidy in embryos are trisomies, in which an individual chromosome is present in triplicate, or monosomies, where only one copy is present, resulting in 47 or 45 chromosomes per cell, respectively. Chromosomes can also be present in multiple copies (tetrasomy, pentasomy, polysomy) or none at all (nullisomy), and more than one chromosome can be affected in the karyotype (double aneuploids, complex aneuploids).

Aneuploidy results from erroneous chromosome segregation during cell division, which can occur during meiosis in gametogenesis or during mitosis in embryonic development. Both meiosis and mitosis are highly complex, coordinated processes that depend on the correct formation of an intricate network of microtubules known as the spindle, responsible for physically moving chromosomal content during cell division. Compromised formation of the spindle can prevent correct segregation of chromosomes or chromatids to daughter cells.

Natural human embryo mortality from fertilization to live birth in normal healthy women is estimated to be no less than 40%–60% [98]. Aneuploidy is common in preimplantation embryos and is thought to be the leading cause of reproductive failure and pregnancy loss in natural conceptions [7,99,100]. Embryos monosomic for any autosome often fail to implant and invariably fail to develop to term because of the insufficient dosage of essential genes. This is also true for the majority of trisomic embryos, which experience excesses in gene dosage. However, trisomies in some autosomes, notably 13, 18, and 21, can result in live births, albeit often with limited survival or lifelong medical ramifications. Sex chromosomes are more permissive of copy number abnormalities, and offspring experience clinical conditions ranging from undetectable to severe.

In IVF, overall some 40% of blastocyst-stage embryos contain aneuploidies, both in natural ovulation and superovulation cycles [101]. The majority of aneuploidies are thought to originate in the oocyte [95,102], and there is a well-documented correlation between maternal age and incidence of aneuploidy both in natural conceptions and in IVF embryos [7]. The higher likelihood of conceiving a Down syndrome fetus with increasing maternal age has long been known [103]. In IVF, the proportion of embryos in a patient's embryo cohort that are aneuploid increases progressively from 30% in women in their early 30s to more than 90% when reaching the age of 44 [14]. A recent large-scale analysis of over 130,000 PGT-A embryos revealed that the incidence of embryos with single chromosome aneuploidies remains relatively constant across ages, but aneuploidies involving two to five different chromosomes become progressively more prevalent with advancing maternal age [104]. Various explanations have been proposed for this correlation. Prolonged exposure to environmental insult, the accumulation of reactive oxygen species (ROS) [105], and/or carbonyl stress that might affect mitochondrial integrity [106] might all result in abnormal spindle formation and aberrant chromosomal segregation during meiosis. Direct observation of compromised meiotic spindles in AMA patients supports this notion [107]. While this renders AMA the leading referral category for PGT-A, the significant presence of aneuploid embryos observed in some younger and donor IVF cycles provides a powerful rationale for PGT-A in all IVF cycles [108].

Segmental Aneuploidy

Contemporary interpretations of aneuploidy in embryology also include segmental losses and gains, where there are deviations in the normal copy number of subchromosomal stretches affecting several megabases (Mb). Such chromosomal abnormalities in embryos were first documented in murine models using classical cytogenetic methods [109]. Most present-day PGT-A platforms are validated to detect partial chromosomal abnormalities of at least 20 Mb. Segmental aneuploidies are mainly believed to originate from mitotic errors during early cell divisions in the forming embryo. This developmental period is associated with weakened cell cycle checkpoints, lax DNA damage repair mechanisms, and double-strand breaks due to rapid proliferation [110,111]. Approximately 16% of IVF-generated blastocysts contain segmental losses or gains. Interestingly, of these segmental aneuploids, only 5% arrive from germ cell−derived errors, largely from the paternal contribution [95].

Identification of segmental aneuploidies during PGT-A is important, as they are present in ~6% of established pregnancies that miscarry, and babies born with such chromosomal errors can experience serious clinical consequences such as seen in Cri-du-chat, Wolf-Hirschhorn, or Jacobson syndromes [112,113].

Chromosomal Mosaicism in Embryos

While the concept of aneuploidy operates on an individual cell level, entire embryos are sometimes referred to as "aneuploid," suggesting that all of the cells present are chromosomally abnormal. Systematic "cell-by-cell" analysis has, however, yet to be performed on a large number of human blastocyst embryos, and thus the prevailing supposition that when the anomaly is a consequence of meiotic errors, then all cells are affected equally still requires validation. In other words, if the aneuploidy is present from the onset of fertilization, the zygote will pass on the chromosomal abnormality to all descendent cells over subsequent cell divisions. As with karyotypically normal embryos, however, a chromosome segregation error could happen during mitosis as a post-zygotic event and mosaicism will arise. A simpler (and thought to be more common) mechanism is where a post-zygotic error arises in a euploid embryo and this attracts the most attention with respect to PGT-A.

Mosaicism was first documented in human embryos with FISH [3,4,52,114]. Since then, a number of different mitotic error mechanisms have been proposed to explain mosaicism: mitotic nondisjunction, anaphase lagging, formation of multinuclei and/or micronuclei, centriole/centrosome dysregulation, and endoreplication [102,115–117]. Mitotic nondisjunction means that sister chromatids of a chromosome are not correctly separated during cell division, resulting in one trisomic and one monosomic daughter cell. Anaphase lagging is an event leading to monosomy in one of the daughter cells at mitosis, because a chromatid does not become incorporated into the nucleus. In mosaic embryos, there is a documented increased incidence of monosomies compared to trisomies, suggesting that anaphase lagging might be the principal mechanism creating mosaicism [12,118,119]. Micronuclei, or small nucleus-like structures, are thought to arise when chromosomal material forms its own nuclear membrane. Since proper kinetochores are absent, the chromosomal content of micronuclei are unable to undergo regulated mitosis, likely resulting in mosaicism in daughter cells [116,120]. Finally, endoreplication without subsequent division could hypothetically result in mosaicism but has not been documented for individual chromosomes, but rather for entire chromosomal complements [115].

Of particular note is so-called "trisomy rescue" (otherwise known as "embryo correction"), where cells lose one of the extra chromosomes that were originally involved in the trisomy. This mechanism can lead to mosaicism but its incidence or precise mode of action is currently not known. This may account for some cases of UPD when the two chromosomes that prevail after the "rescue event" are derived from the same parent. UPD is seen in newborns at an incidence of 1 in 3500 [121].

Evidence from a mouse model for aneuploidy indicates that meiotically induced aneuploidy might trigger downstream mitotic events. Using synaptonemal complex protein 3 (SYCP3)-null mice, which experience chromosomal missegregation during meiosis, a study has shown that aneuploid embryos become cytologically unstable, resulting in a rapid evolution of mosaicism and early embryonic death by apoptosis independent of the p53 mechanism [122,123].

In general, it is thought that cleavage-stage embryos are more prone to be mosaic than blastocysts [124]. A systematic review of FISH studies indicated that 75% of cleavage-stage embryos were mosaic [125], later confirmed by comprehensive chromosome screening techniques on good quality IVF cleavage-stage embryos from young patients (<35 years) reporting a 70% mosaicism rate [126]. During the first cell divisions, the embryonic genome is largely inactive, meaning that cell cycle progression is solely regulated by maternally derived factors independent of transcription. A dampened governance of the cell cycle might result in increased mitotic errors, explaining the common occurrence of mosaicism at the cleavage stage [127]. This could in turn explain why cleavage-stage PGT-A, in which a single cell is analyzed, has been largely considered ineffective [15], although some RCTs have shown tangible benefits in some patient groups [46,128].

Though not as common, blastocyst-stage mosaicism has also been demonstrated with FISH analysis of fixed whole embryos, and mosaic mixes have been documented in the inner cell mass (ICM) as well as trophectoderm (TE) tissues [129,130]. Blastocyst-stage mosaicism might be less prevalent because some mosaic embryos might arrest during development [127], especially in cases with high aneuploid cell load. Data from mouse experiments support this notion, as it was shown that chimeric embryos composed of different ratios of euploid and aneuploid cells have different viability. In these studies, transferred embryos with a ratio of 1:3 euploid-to-aneuploid cells never resulted in a live birth, whereas those with a 1:1 ratio had a 50% chance of coming to term [131]. Analysis of cell proliferation and death indicated that in surviving embryos, euploid cells tended to outcompete aneuploid ones. This means that mosaic embryos might be able to self-correct and become entirely euploid, offering an alternative explanation for why less mosaicism is observed at the blastocyst stage compared to earlier stages [127]. Moreover, mosaicism rate is reported as less than 1%–2% in viable pregnancies [132], suggesting other mechanisms are still at play after implantation.

Whether a mosaic embryo is capable of implanting and its subsequent clinical fate depend on a variety of factors. These include the timing of the segregational error, the proportion and the lineage of the embryo that has been affected, and the type of abnormalities and the chromosome(s) involved [97,133]. Conceptually, an embryo would be predicted to be less severely affected when the error occurs at later stages of development, most likely resulting in confined mosaicism [133]. This is particularly relevant in that a meiotic error, or one in the very earliest cleavage divisions, would most likely be the most clinically significant, as it would affect the majority of cells in the embryo. Whereas if the mitotic error occurs later in development, when cell lineages have already segregated, the clinical consequences might be different. For example, confined placental mosaicism (CPM), in which aneuploid cells are confined to the placenta, can lead to intrauterine growth retardation or placental insufficiency [134].

The incidence of mitotically derived mosaicism in embryos does not increase with maternal age, in contrast to meiotic aneuploidy where there is a far clearer age correlation [54,125–127]. This indicates that age-related factors leading to increased meiotic errors do not play a role in mitotic errors, which appear to have a uniform baseline error rate across patients. This concept is markedly at odds with the notion that errors in mitosis are more common in an already aneuploid setting due to a previous meiotic event. Such discrepant hypotheses remain to be resolved as we continue to learn more about the biological mechanisms of mosaicism. Indeed, maternally derived factors are likely not solely responsible for the creation of mosaic embryos. As centrosomes are paternally inherited and are responsible for spindle formation during mitosis, there is a likely paternal contribution to mosaicism formation. In fact, disruption of centrosomes increases mosaicism rates in embryos [135]. Additionally, it is thought that laboratory procedures might influence rates of mosaicism, as incidence of mosaic embryos varies greatly between IVF centers [81]. Culture conditions, ovarian hyperstimulation strategies, and biopsy techniques (including excessive use of laser thermal ablation) have all been hypothesized to have a significant influence on the measured rates of mosaicism, as they might influence the chance of aberrant mitosis or compromised biopsy material [136]. Rates of mosaicism might therefore be a key performance indicator for quality assurance in IVF laboratories. The reported proportion of IVF embryos that are classified as mosaic has varied widely, ranging from under 4% to over 90% [137]. The estimation depends heavily on various factors such as embryo characteristics, biopsy techniques, PGT-A platform employed, and thresholds used to define mosaicism. The clinical challenges that this brings are dealt with in the next section.

Mosaicism Detection and Its Clinical Implications

A PGT-A platform designed to provide mosaicism information should be sensitive enough to detect mosaicism in 5–10 cells. Several laboratories using NGS have performed euploid/aneuploid-mixing experiments using cell lines with different known aneuploidies, resulting in profiles consistent with mosaicism [82,83,138–140]. Analysis is usually sensitive enough to estimate the percentage of aneuploid cells in the biopsy and characterize as segmental, monosomy, trisomy, or multiple chromosomes. PGDIS [141] and CoGEN [142] have published position statements defining mosaicism in PGT-A. These were based on initial validation studies proposing that karyotype profiles deviating from disomic values by <20% should be treated as normal, those with >80% as abnormal, and the remaining ones between 20%–80% as mosaic [81,143]. It must be noted, however, that technical artifacts can also result in profiles with intermediate values that errantly suggest mosaicism [137,144]. Irregularities of the WGA procedure and S-phase artifacts (potential intermediate conformations of DNA during the synthesis phase of the cell cycle) can affect the output of the process. Validation and recurrent quality control of the PGT-A platform used are therefore paramount, and individual low-quality PGT-A results should be interpreted carefully.

Studies from different groups have repeatedly shown that blastocysts classified as mosaic with PGT-A possess a distinct set of clinical outcomes compared to those classified as fully euploid [82,138,145,146]. This suggests that a diagnosis of mosaicism is not just an artifact of PGT-A, but rather a reflection of a biological phenomenon. Even blastocysts categorized as "low mosaics" have poorer outcomes than the euploid group, indicating they are not merely euploids wrongly classified as mosaics because of technical noise.

The first report of mosaic embryo transfers appeared in 2015 and showed that such embryos could implant and lead to babies that appeared normal by routine medical examination at birth [147]. Since then, there have been more than 400 embryos classified as mosaic that have been transferred, leading to over 50 births. So far there have been no reports of compromised newborns. The inevitable questions are: Are children born from mosaic embryo transfers truly "healthy?" And if so, how is it that they are not affected in any appreciable way? These questions might be difficult to answer. While there have been no reports of obvious symptoms, more subtle conditions might yet be uncovered or could appear later in life for those children. To date there have not been any studies thoroughly investigating whether a higher-than-usual load of abnormal cells is found in various tissues of infants that were diagnosed as mosaic at the blastocyst stage. Furthermore, nothing is known about potential epigenetic or transcriptomic consequences of mosaicism in embryos.

The phenomenon of mosaicism poses an additional challenge to PGT-A. Looking at the blastocyst as a whole, mosaicism could lead to false PGT-A results even when uniform aneuploidy or euploidy is diagnosed in the TE biopsy. Since the TE biopsy is taken from a random sample in the tissue, it is possible that the whole collection of cells in the biopsy has a different chromosomal makeup than parts or the entire remaining embryo. Studies have explored the incidence of such a situation by analyzing serial biopsies in individual blastocysts and determining rates of concordance [148]. The most recent reports, which analyze the various TE and ICM biopsies by NGS, demonstrate that non-mosaic, uniform aneuploidies or euploidies detected in a TE biopsy are excellent predictors of the chromosomal status in the remaining embryo [140,149]. For whole-chromosome aneuploidies, a clinical TE biopsy is 96.4% predictive of aneuploidy in the ICM. Segmental aneuploidies appear to be less concordant between serial biopsies, but this needs to be confirmed in larger datasets [149,150]. The incidence of segmental aneuploidies is unrelated to maternal age [104], just as is the case with embryos in the mosaic category. Intrablastocyst mosaicism is also unsurprisingly a poor predictor of the karyotype content of the remaining cells in the conceptus [82,140].

The position statements of PGDIS and CoGEN recommend that if no euploid embryos are available, patients may opt to transfer an embryo classified as mosaic, prioritizing certain chromosomes. In such cases, mosaic trisomies in chromosomes X, Y, 13, 18, and 21, and monosomies in X are typically not recommended for transfer, as those aneuploidies are viable. Aneuploidies in chromosomes 14 and 15 are also considered problematic, since trisomy or monosomy rescue could lead to UPD, known to have clinical consequences in the mentioned chromosomes. Trisomies in chromosomes 2, 7, and 16 can lead to intrauterine growth retardation, so mosaicisms affecting those chromosomes are low priority for transfer.

The position statements also recommend follow-up with the patient if pregnancy is established, including noninvasive prenatal testing (NIPT), chorionic villus sampling (CVS), or, preferably, amniocentesis (which tests cells derived from fetal rather than placental tissue). A study on the occurrence of mosaicism in products of conception has produced some guidelines for prioritizing mosaic embryos based on the likelihood of mosaicism in individual chromosomes to result in miscarriages [151,152]. The currently published reports on mosaic embryo transfers, although numerous, are individually quite limited in sample size, with none surpassing 143 transferred embryos. This has led to some contradictory observations; for example, one study claiming that increasing level of mosaicism (the percentage of aneuploid cells present in the TE biopsy) adversely affects clinical outcomes [146], and another refuting that finding [82]. Evidence-based guidelines will solidify over the next years with increasing sample sizes and comprehensive analyses.

Mitochondrial DNA and Its Role in PGT-A

During PGT-A, aside from the analysis of nuclear DNA content, cellular biopsies can be evaluated for mitochondrial DNA (mtDNA) load. mtDNA is a circular nucleic acid molecule present in each human cell as multiple copies. Two groups published independent studies in 2015 indicating that high mtDNA content per cell correlated with poor embryo viability [153,154]. They described a threshold of mtDNA copy number that if surpassed always led to failed implantation upon transfer. One of the groups published two additional studies supporting the findings, although noting that some clinics did not generate blastocysts with a greatly elevated mtDNA copy number [155,156]. Publications from other laboratories could not reproduce the results [157–160]. Noting that vastly different mtDNA quantitation methods were used between studies, it was suggested that technical variability could have caused the contradictory observations. Guidelines were hence proposed with the intent to standardize mtDNA copy number analysis during PGT-A [161]. Recently, a study adhering to those guidelines reported the implantation of blastocysts with a highly elevated mtDNA copy number, which led to subsequent healthy births [162]. The use of mtDNA copy number assessment as a routine PGT-A "add-on" to further rank euploid embryos has therefore largely been discredited. Whether it will find some use in particular settings remains to be determined.

The Prospects for Noninvasive PGT-A

While removing 5–10 cells of the TE in a biopsy for PGT-A has largely been shown to be inconsequential to the viability of a blastocyst [35], the physical process of collecting a TE biopsy can be damaging to the embryo if done incorrectly. It is also a cumbersome technique that requires highly skilled embryologists. As a result, there is great interest in developing methods of noninvasive PGT-A (niPGT-A).

Blastocentesis

Blastocentesis refers to the extraction of blastocoelic fluid for subsequent analysis. Blastocoelic fluid is known to contain DNA originating from embryonic cells as well as proteins involved in embryonic development [163,164]. In this technique, blastocoelic fluid is aspirated through an ICSI pipette, a process of limited invasiveness. Each blastocyst yields approximately 0.01 μL blastocele fluid (BF), which is subsequently amplified by WGA [165]. In a study performed to investigate the potential of blastocoelic fluid as a diagnostic sample, the DNA could be obtained in 82% of the sampled fluids; 97.1% of the diagnosis results were in concordance with trophectoderm cells [166]. Other studies have failed to replicate these high rates of concordance, as highlighted in a report in which only 40% of blastocoelic fluid cases reflected the ploidy of the embryo [139]. Recently, it was shown that aneuploid embryos contained significantly higher overall quantities of DNA than euploids in the blastocoelic fluid, likely due to higher rates of apoptosis in aneuploid cells [167]. This could lead to a minimally invasive PGT-A method that simply quantifies DNA amounts in the BF. Future studies with large sample sizes will be needed to validate this proposed method.

Analysis of Spent Culture Medium

True niPGT-A would mean letting the embryo grow undisturbed until vitrification or fresh transfer and still somehow gaining knowledge on its viability. Efforts are currently focused on analysis of spent medium (SM) for biomarkers predictive of embryo state and clinical outcome, including DNA, RNA, protein, metabolites, and exosomes. Initial efforts mainly focused on amino acid analysis in the SM but showed limited potential for routine application [168,169].

More recently, research has focused on DNA in SM. Cell-free DNA (cfDNA) derived from the embryo is present in the SM through processes that are yet to be understood but likely involve apoptosis and other cell death pathways or DNA-based signaling. Whether the cfDNA is of sufficient quantity and quality to reliably be analyzed and whether it is truly reflective of the embryo's karyotype are questions currently being investigated in a fast-moving field. A flurry of recent reports using state-of-the-art NGS platforms observed ploidy concordance rates between SM and blastocyst cells in the 80%–95% range [170–174]. Nevertheless, it is crucial to note that the SM analyzed in those studies might not have been pristine; in every instance the authors performed some procedure that could artificially increase the abundance of cfDNA in the SM, such as assisted hatching, freeze-thaw cycle, or invasively isolating a TE biopsy before collecting the SM. Only one recent publication has avoided such confounding procedures altogether in addition to having been conducted blindly and prospectively, and it reports a 78.7% concordance rate for ploidy and sex between SM and TE [175]. Various efforts are underway to modify the culture methods, spent medium collection method, WGA chemistry, and NGS process and analysis to continue inching up the concordance rates. It is important to note that 100% concordance between SM and TE may not be realistic, and this could be because SM turns out to be a more accurate representation of the embryonic genotype for reasons that are not yet well understood. Better rates of concordance are observed in embryos cultured to embryonic day 6 or 7 over those cultured only to day 5, but the most successful blastocysts are typically those vitrified on developmental day 5 [176]. Maternal DNA contamination in the medium, mainly through cumulus cells, can affect the ploidy as well as the sex in the SM PGT-A results [177].

How Sensitive Is niPGT-A Regarding Segmental Deletions/Duplications, and Mosaicism?

Interestingly, niPGT might not need to be regarded as a one-to-one substitute of TE biopsy-based PGT-A. It might serve as a low-resolution screening tool for laboratories that choose not to perform TE biopsy, or it can be done in parallel with the TE analysis. One study shows that concordant euploid in paired SM-TE samples predicts better likelihood of implantation for an embryo than when its TE biopsy is euploid but its SM shows aneuploidy (52.9% vs. 16.7%, respectively) [175]. Recently a new kit specifically for niPGT-A has been released by Perkin Elmer, and we await large studies in its sensitivity.

Owing to the uncertainty and confusion generated by the detection and reporting in the absence of clinical data, some might argue that looking at the content of SM may be a better evaluation of the embryo than an individual trophectoderm biopsy. This is a rapidly evolving field and, if successful, will revolutionize the PGT-A landscape.

Morphokinetics and Time-Lapse for Aneuploidy Detection

Another avenue being explored to evaluate embryos in a noninvasive way is the continuous monitoring via time-lapse imaging technology during culture. Some studies have indicated that embryos exhibit different kinetic behavior in cell division patterns according to their ploidy [178–181]. Other reports have refuted that claim [182–184]. Another set of studies has explored the correlation between morphokinetic patterns and implantation potential, rather than strict ploidy state, with promising results [185,186].

Time-lapse monitoring must not necessarily need to replace PGT-A altogether but might instead offer an added benefit, as the two technologies can be performed in parallel. For instance, morphokinetic patterns might help rank embryos classified by PGT-A as euploid with highest chance of implantation and decreased chance of miscarriage, as has recently been attempted with some success [84,187]. Future work will need to address this point.

Conclusions

Despite the sometimes-heated controversy regarding the efficacy of PGT-A, it is a technology that is likely here to stay (Figure 3.1). The availability of higher-resolution platforms has shifted the conversation beyond ploidy, and arguably expanded the utility of the test. As testing platforms continue to improve, additional information will likely become available regarding the genomic, transcriptomic, and epigenetic status of an embryo. As we make sense of this additional information and its relationship to downstream outcomes, one can envision a world where every IVF embryo undergoes some form of PGT. A single test may offer a comprehensive picture regarding the absolute health of an embryo and that of the resultant fetus, offering additional refinements to the science of embryo selection. Perhaps the "-A" in PGT-A will become obsolete, as the lines between PGT-M/-SR/-P and -A will be blurred.

As these technologies allow us to gain invaluable insights into early human embryonic development, we may also gain insight into the populations we treat. Combining our findings with those from companies like Previvo Genetics, Inc. that have developed techniques to recover embryos conceived *in vivo* in order to perform PGT may help further the discussions of the dissonance between *in vitro* and *in vivo* conceptuses, and fertile vs. infertile populations, potentially leading to improvements in the ways we perform IVF and treat different subsets of patients.

For the foreseeable future, however, given an aging population and trends toward reproduction later in life, the demand for status quo PGT-A is likely to continue to increase as female age is one of the significant genetic problems facing reproduction. It is, of course, never acceptable to be reckless in the application of any medical genetic test, especially one as high stakes as PGT that determines the fate of embryos, and ongoing RCTs are crucial checkpoints—*primum non nocere*. However, refusal to lend at least some credibility to its potential seems equally as reckless, potentially causing patients to confer significant physiological, financial, and psychological stress due to miscarriages, failed implantation, and

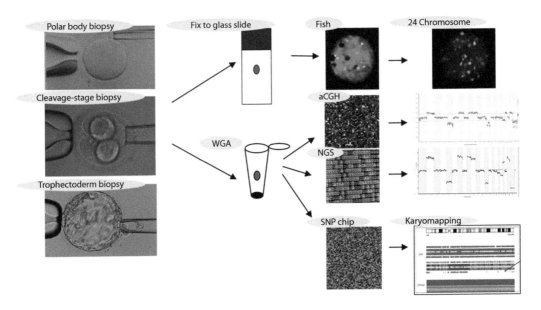

FIGURE 3.1 Overview of PGT-A indicating biopsy and diagnostic techniques.

delays in establishing a viable pregnancy. A reminder that benefits from a test as unique as PGT-A may be more complex than what previous and current RCTs are after, and perhaps additional criteria need to be included in the discussion and quantification of its efficacy.

Declaration of Interests

Three of the authors (AV, CO, AT) are employed by private IVF and/or diagnostic companies that could potentially benefit from the use of PGT-A.

REFERENCES

1. Edwards RG, Gardner RL. Sexing of live rabbit blastocysts. *Nature.* 1967;214:576–7.
2. Handyside AH, Kontogianni EH, Hardy K, Winston RM. Pregnancies from biopsied human preimplantation embryos sexed by Y-specific DNA amplification. *Nature.* 1990;344:768–70.
3. Griffin DK, Wilton LJ, Handyside AH, Winston RM, Delhanty JD. Dual fluorescent in situ hybridisation for simultaneous detection of X and Y chromosome-specific probes for the sexing of human preimplantation embryonic nuclei. *Hum Genet.* 1992;89:18–22.
4. Griffin DK, Wilton LJ, Handyside AH, Atkinson GH, Winston RM, Delhanty JD. Diagnosis of sex in preimplantation embryos by fluorescent in situ hybridisation. *BMJ.* 1993;306:1382.
5. Schrurs BM, Winston RM, Handyside AH. Preimplantation diagnosis of aneuploidy using fluorescent in-situ hybridization: Evaluation using a chromosome 18-specific probe. *Hum Reprod.* 1993;8:296–301.
6. Munne S, Lee A, Rosenwaks Z, Grifo J, Cohen J. Diagnosis of major chromosome aneuploidies in human preimplantation embryos. *Hum Reprod.* 1993;8:2185–91.
7. Hassold T, Hunt P. To err (meiotically) is human: The genesis of human aneuploidy. *Nat Rev Genet.* 2001;2:280–91.
8. Findikli N et al. Embryo aneuploidy screening for repeated implantation failure and unexplained recurrent miscarriage. *Reprod Biomed Online.* 2006;13:38–46.
9. Kahraman S et al. Preliminary FISH studies on spermatozoa and embryos in patients with variable degrees of teratozoospermia and a history of poor prognosis. *Reprod Biomed Online.* 2006;12:752–61.
10. Coates A et al. Use of suboptimal sperm increases the risk of aneuploidy of the sex chromosomes in preimplantation blastocyst embryos. *Fertil Steril.* 2015;104:866–72.
11. Ioannou D, Meershoek EJ, Thornhill AR, Ellis M, Griffin DK. Multicolour interphase cytogenetics: 24 chromosome probes, 6 colours, 4 layers. *Mol Cell Probes.* 2011;25:199–205.
12. Ioannou D et al. Twenty-four chromosome FISH in human IVF embryos reveals patterns of post-zygotic chromosome segregation and nuclear organisation. *Chromosome Res.* 2012;20:447–60.
13. Munne S, Fragouli E, Colls P, Katz-Jaffe M, Schoolcraft W, Wells D. Improved detection of aneuploid blastocysts using a new 12-chromosome FISH test. *Reprod Biomed Online.* 2010;20:92–7.
14. Franasiak JM et al. The nature of aneuploidy with increasing age of the female partner: A review of 15,169 consecutive trophectoderm biopsies evaluated with comprehensive chromosomal screening. *Fertil Steril.* 2014;101:656–63 e1.
15. Mastenbroek S et al. In vitro fertilization with preimplantation genetic screening. *N Engl J Med.* 2007;357:9–17.
16. Twisk M et al. No beneficial effect of preimplantation genetic screening in women of advanced maternal age with a high risk for embryonic aneuploidy. *Hum Reprod.* 2008;23:2813–7.
17. Harper JC et al. The ESHRE PGD Consortium: 10 years of data collection. *Hum Reprod Update.* 2012;18:234–47.
18. Kuliev A, Rechitsky S. Preimplantation genetic testing: Current challenges and future prospects. *Expert Rev Mol Diagn.* 2017;17:1071–88.
19. Munne S et al. Preimplantation genetic testing for aneuploidy versus morphology as selection criteria for single frozen-thawed embryo transfer in good-prognosis patients: A multicenter randomized clinical trial. *Fertil Steril.* 2019;112(6):1071–9.
20. Verlinsky Y, Ginsberg N, Lifchez A, Valle J, Moise J, Strom CM. Analysis of the first polar body: Preconception genetic diagnosis. *Hum Reprod.* 1990;5:826–9.

21. Magli MC et al. Polar body array CGH for prediction of the status of the corresponding oocyte. Part II: Technical aspects. *Hum Reprod.* 2011;26:3181–5.

22. Geraedts J et al. What next for preimplantation genetic screening? A polar body approach! *Hum Reprod* 2010;25:575–7.

23. Geraedts J et al. Polar body array CGH for prediction of the status of the corresponding oocyte. Part I: Clinical results. *Hum Reprod.* 2011;26:3173–80.

24. Hardarson T et al. Preimplantation genetic screening in women of advanced maternal age caused a decrease in clinical pregnancy rate: A randomized controlled trial. *Hum Reprod.* 2008;23:2806–12.

25. Fishel S et al. Live birth after polar body array comparative genomic hybridization prediction of embryo ploidy-the future of IVF? *Fertil Steril.* 2010;93:1006.e7–10.

26. Capalbo A et al. Sequential comprehensive chromosome analysis on polar bodies, blastomeres and trophoblast: Insights into female meiotic errors and chromosomal segregation in the preimplantation window of embryo development. *Hum Reprod.* 2013;28:509–18.

27. Salvaggio CN, Forman EJ, Garnsey HM, Treff NR, Scott RT Jr. Polar body based aneuploidy screening is poorly predictive of embryo ploidy and reproductive potential. *J Assist Reprod Genet.* 2014;31:1221–6.

28. Forman EJ et al. Embryos whose polar bodies contain isolated reciprocal chromosome aneuploidy are almost always euploid. *Hum Reprod.* 2013;28:502–8.

29. Feichtinger M et al. Correction: Increasing live birth rate by preimplantation genetic screening of pooled polar bodies using array comparative genomic hybridization. *PLOS ONE.* 2015;10:e0133334.

30. Verpoest W et al. Preimplantation genetic testing for aneuploidy by microarray analysis of polar bodies in advanced maternal age: A randomized clinical trial. *Hum Reprod.* 2018;33:1767–76.

31. Brown S. Still in highESTEEM. Focus on Reproduction - ESHRE Magazine Blog. https://focusonreproduction.eu (accessed July 4, 2017).

32. Cohen J, Wells D, Munne S. Removal of 2 cells from cleavage stage embryos is likely to reduce the efficacy of chromosomal tests that are used to enhance implantation rates. *Fertil Steril.* 2007;87:496–503.

33. Gianaroli L et al. The beneficial effects of preimplantation genetic diagnosis for aneuploidy support extensive clinical application. *Reprod Biomed Online.* 2005;10:633–40.

34. Schoolcraft WB, Katz-Jaffe MG, Stevens J, Rawlins M, Munne S. Preimplantation aneuploidy testing for infertile patients of advanced maternal age: A randomized prospective trial. *Fertil Steril.* 2009;92:157–62.

35. Scott RT Jr., Upham KM, Forman EJ, Zhao T, Treff NR. Cleavage-stage biopsy significantly impairs human embryonic implantation potential while blastocyst biopsy does not: A randomized and paired clinical trial. *Fertil Steril.* 2013;100:624–30.

36. Duncan FE, Stein P, Williams CJ, Schultz RM. The effect of blastomere biopsy on preimplantation mouse embryo development and global gene expression. *Fertil Steril.* 2009;91:1462–5.

37. Kirkegaard K, Hindkjaer JJ, Ingerslev HJ. Human embryonic development after blastomere removal: A time-lapse analysis. *Hum Reprod.* 2012;27:97–105.

38. McArthur SJ, Leigh D, Marshall JT, de Boer KA, Jansen RP. Pregnancies and live births after trophectoderm biopsy and preimplantation genetic testing of human blastocysts. *Fertil Steril.* 2005;84:1628–36.

39. Forman EJ, Ferry KM, Gueye N-A, Smith RD, Stevens J, Scott RT Jr. Trophectoderm biopsy for single-gene disorder preimplantation genetic diagnosis (PGD) is significantly more reliable than day 3 blastomere biopsy. *Fertil Steril.* 2011;96:S222.

40. Kokkali G et al. Blastocyst biopsy versus cleavage stage biopsy and blastocyst transfer for preimplantation genetic diagnosis of beta-thalassaemia: A pilot study. *Hum Reprod.* 2007;22:1443–9.

41. Forman EJ et al. In vitro fertilization with single euploid blastocyst transfer: A randomized controlled trial. *Fertil Steril.* 2013;100:100–7 e1.

42. Ubaldi FM et al. Reduction of multiple pregnancies in the advanced maternal age population after implementation of an elective single embryo transfer policy coupled with enhanced embryo selection: Pre- and post-intervention study. *Hum Reprod.* 2015;30:2097–106.

43. Capalbo A et al. Consistent and reproducible outcomes of blastocyst biopsy and aneuploidy screening across different biopsy practitioners: A multicentre study involving 2586 embryo biopsies. *Hum Reprod.* 2016;31:199–208.

44. Yang Z et al. Selection of single blastocysts for fresh transfer via standard morphology assessment alone and with array CGH for good prognosis IVF patients: Results from a randomized pilot study. *Mol Cytogenet* 2012;5:24.

45. Scott RT Jr. et al. Blastocyst biopsy with comprehensive chromosome screening and fresh embryo transfer significantly increases in vitro fertilization implantation and delivery rates: A randomized controlled trial. *Fertil Steril.* 2013;100:697–703.

46. Rubio C et al. In vitro fertilization with preimplantation genetic diagnosis for aneuploidies in advanced maternal age: A randomized, controlled study. *Fertil Steril.* 2017;107:1122–9.

47. Cobo A, de los Santos MJ, Castello D, Gamiz P, Campos P, Remohi J. Outcomes of vitrified early cleavage-stage and blastocyst-stage embryos in a cryopreservation program: Evaluation of 3,150 warming cycles. *Fertil Steril.* 2012;98:1138–46 e1.

48. Roy TK, Bradley CK, Bowman MC, McArthur SJ. Single-embryo transfer of vitrified-warmed blastocysts yields equivalent live-birth rates and improved neonatal outcomes compared with fresh transfers. *Fertil Steril.* 2014;101:1294–301.

49. Koot YE et al. An endometrial gene expression signature accurately predicts recurrent implantation failure after IVF. *Sci Rep.* 2016;6:19411.

50. Mahajan N. Endometrial receptivity array: Clinical application. *J Hum Reprod Sci* 2015;8:121–9.

51. Altmae S et al. Endometrial transcriptome analysis indicates superiority of natural over artificial cycles in recurrent implantation failure patients undergoing frozen embryo transfer. *Reprod Biomed Online.* 2016;32:597–613.

52. Delhanty JD et al. Detection of aneuploidy and chromosomal mosaicism in human embryos during preimplantation sex determination by fluorescent in situ hybridisation, (FISH). *Hum Mol Genet.* 1993;2:1183–5.

53. Munne S, Sandalinas M, Magli C, Gianaroli L, Cohen J, Warburton D. Increased rate of aneuploid embryos in young women with previous aneuploid conceptions. *Prenat Diagn.* 2004;24:638–43.

54. Turner K, Fowler K, Fonseka G, Griffin D, Ioannou D. Multicolor detection of every chromosome as a means of detecting mosaicism and nuclear organization in human embryonic nuclei. *Panminerva Med.* 2016;58:175–90.

55. Deleye L et al. Whole genome amplification with SurePlex results in better copy number alteration detection using sequencing data compared to the MALBAC method. *Sci Rep.* 2015;5:11711.

56. Blagodatskikh KA et al. Improved DOP-PCR (iDOP-PCR): A robust and simple WGA method for efficient amplification of low copy number genomic DNA. *PLOS ONE.* 2017;12:e0184507.

57. Babayan A et al. Comparative study of whole genome amplification and next generation sequencing performance of single cancer cells. *Oncotarget.* 2017;8:56066–80.

58. Chen M et al. Comparison of multiple displacement amplification (MDA) and multiple annealing and looping-based amplification cycles (MALBAC) in single-cell sequencing. *PLOS ONE.* 2014;9:e114520.

59. Deleye L, Tilleman L, Vander Plaetsen AS, Cornelis S, Deforce D, Van Nieuwerburgh F. Performance of four modern whole genome amplification methods for copy number variant detection in single cells. *Sci Rep.* 2017;7:3422.

60. Li W et al. The mutation-free embryo for in vitro fertilization selected by MALBAC-PGD resulted in a healthy live birth from a family carrying PKD 1 mutation. *J Assist Reprod Genet.* 2017;34:1653–8.

61. Kallioniemi A et al. Comparative genomic hybridization for molecular cytogenetic analysis of solid tumors. *Science.* 1992;258:818–21.

62. Spelcher MR et al. Molecular cytogenetic analysis of formalin-fixed, paraffin-embedded solid tumors by comparative genomic hybridization after universal DNA-amplification. *Hum Mol Genet.* 1993;2:1907–14.

63. Forozan F, Karhu R, Kononen J, Kallioniemi A, Kallioniemi O-P. Genome screening by comparative genomic hybridization. *Trends Genet.* 1997;13:405–9.

64. Wilton L. Preimplantation genetic diagnosis and chromosome analysis of blastomeres using comparative genomic hybridization. *Hum Reprod Update.* 2005;11:33–41.

65. Wells D, Escudero T, Levy B, Hirschhorn K, Delhanty JD, Munne S. First clinical application of comparative genomic hybridization and polar body testing for preimplantation genetic diagnosis of aneuploidy. *Fertil Steril.* 2002;78:543–9.

66. Kirchhoff M, Gerdes T, Rose H, Maahr J, Ottesen AM, Lundsteen C. Detection of chromosomal gains and losses in comparative genomic hybridization analysis based on standard reference intervals. *Cytometry.* 1998;31:163–73.

67. Lichter P, Joos S, Bentz M, Lampel S. Comparative genomic hybridization: Uses and limitations. *Semin Hematol.* 2000 Oct;37(4):348–57.

68. De Ravel TJ, Devriendt K, Fryns J-P, Vermeesch JR. What's new in karyotyping? The move towards array comparative genomic hybridisation (CGH). *Eur J Pediatr.* 2007;166:637–43.

69. Le Caignec C et al. Single-cell chromosomal imbalances detection by array CGH. *Nucleic Acids Res.* 2006;34:e68.

70. Traversa MV, Marshall J, McArthur S, Leigh D. The genetic screening of preimplantation embryos by comparative genomic hybridisation. *Reprod Biol.* 2011;11 Suppl 3:51–60.

71. Vanneste E et al. What next for preimplantation genetic screening? High mitotic chromosome instability rate provides the biological basis for the low success rate. *Hum Reprod.* 2009;24:2679–82.

72. Fiorentino F et al. PGD for reciprocal and Robertsonian translocations using array comparative genomic hybridization. *Hum Reprod.* 2011;26:1925–35.

73. Johnson DS et al. Preclinical validation of a microarray method for full molecular karyotyping of blastomeres in a 24-h protocol. *Hum Reprod.* 2010;25:1066–75.

74. Keltz MD et al. Preimplantation genetic screening (PGS) with Comparative genomic hybridization (CGH) following day 3 single cell blastomere biopsy markedly improves IVF outcomes while lowering multiple pregnancies and miscarriages. *J Assist Reprod Genet.* 2013;30:1333–9.

75. Mamas T, Gordon A, Brown A, Harper J, Sengupta S. Detection of aneuploidy by array comparative genomic hybridization using cell lines to mimic a mosaic trophectoderm biopsy. *Fertil Steril.* 2012;97:943–7.

76. Fiorentino F et al. Development and validation of a next-generation sequencing-based protocol for 24-chromosome aneuploidy screening of embryos. *Fertil Steril.* 2014;101:1375–82.

77. Wells D et al. Clinical utilisation of a rapid low-pass whole genome sequencing technique for the diagnosis of aneuploidy in human embryos prior to implantation. *J Med Genet.* 2014;51:553–62.

78. Zheng H, Jin H, Liu L, Liu J, Wang WH. Application of next-generation sequencing for 24-chromosome aneuploidy screening of human preimplantation embryos. *Mol Cytogenet* 2015;8:38.

79. Knapp M, Stiller M, Meyer M. Generating barcoded libraries for multiplex high-throughput sequencing. *Methods Mol Biol.* 2012;840:155–70.

80. Treff NR et al. Validation of concurrent preimplantation genetic testing for polygenic and monogenic disorders, structural rearrangements, and whole and segmental chromosome aneuploidy with a single universal platform. *Eur J Med Genet.* 2019;62:103647.

81. Munne S, Wells D. Detection of mosaicism at blastocyst stage with the use of high-resolution next-generation sequencing. *Fertil Steril.* 2017;107:1085–91.

82. Victor AR et al. One hundred mosaic embryos transferred prospectively in a single clinic: Exploring when and why they result in healthy pregnancies. *Fertil Steril.* 2019;111:280–93.

83. Maxwell SM et al. Why do euploid embryos miscarry? A case-control study comparing the rate of aneuploidy within presumed euploid embryos that resulted in miscarriage or live birth using next-generation sequencing. *Fertil Steril.* 2016;106:1414–9 e5.

84. Lee CI et al. Embryo morphokinetics is potentially associated with clinical outcomes of single-embryo transfers in preimplantation genetic testing for aneuploidy cycles. *Reprod Biomed Online.* 2019;39:569–79.

85. Treff NR, Scott RT. Four-hour quantitative real-time polymerase chain reaction–based comprehensive chromosome screening and accumulating evidence of accuracy, safety, predictive value, and clinical efficacy. *Fertil Steril.* 2013b;99:1049–53.

86. Treff NR, Tao X, Ferry KM, Su J, Taylor D, Scott RT. Development and validation of an accurate quantitative real-time polymerase chain reaction-based assay for human blastocyst comprehensive chromosomal aneuploidy screening. *Fertil Steril.* 2012;97:819–24. e2.

87. Dahdouh EM et al. Technical update: Preimplantation genetic diagnosis and screening. *J Obstet Gynaecol Can.* 2015;37:451–63.

88. Treff NR, Tao X, Ferry KM, Su J, Taylor D, Scott RT Jr. Development and validation of an accurate quantitative real-time polymerase chain reaction-based assay for human blastocyst comprehensive chromosomal aneuploidy screening. *Fertil Steril.* 2012;97:819–24.

89. Dahdouh EM et al. Technical update: Preimplantation genetic diagnosis and screening. *Obstet Gynecol Surv.* 2015;70:557–8.

90. LaFramboise T. Single nucleotide polymorphism arrays: A decade of biological, computational and technological advances. *Nucleic Acids Res.* 2009;37:4181–93.

91. Treff NR, Northrop LE, Kasabwala K, Su J, Levy B, Scott RT. Single nucleotide polymorphism microarray–based concurrent screening of 24-chromosome aneuploidy and unbalanced translocations in preimplantation human embryos. *Fertil Steril.* 2011;95:1606–12. e2.

92. Handyside AH. Live births following karyomapping - a "key" milestone in the development of preimplantation genetic diagnosis. *Reprod Biomed Online.* 2015;31:307–8.

93. Rabinowitz M et al. Origins and rates of aneuploidy in human blastomeres. *Fertil Steril.* 2012;97:395–401.

94. Natesan SA et al. Genome-wide karyomapping accurately identifies the inheritance of single-gene defects in human preimplantation embryos in vitro. *Genet Med.* 2014;16(11):838–45.

95. Kubicek D et al. Incidence and origin of meiotic whole and segmental chromosomal aneuploidies detected by karyomapping. *Reprod Biomed Online.* 2019;38:330–9.

96. Zamani Esteki M et al. Concurrent whole-genome haplotyping and copy-number profiling of single cells. *Am J Hum Genet.* 2015;96:894–912.

97. Wolstenholme J. Confined placental mosaicism for trisomies 2, 3, 7, 8, 9, 16, and 22: Their incidence, likely origins, and mechanisms for cell lineage compartmentalization. *Prenat Diagn.* 1996;16:511–24.

98. Jarvis GE. Estimating limits for natural human embryo mortality. *F1000Res.* 2016;5:2083.

99. Benkhalifa M et al. Array comparative genomic hybridization profiling of first-trimester spontaneous abortions that fail to grow in vitro. *Prenat Diagn.* 2005;25:894–900.

100. Hodes-Wertz B et al. Idiopathic recurrent miscarriage is caused mostly by aneuploid embryos. *Fertil Steril.* 2012;98:675–80.

101. Munne S. Preimplantation genetic diagnosis for aneuploidy and translocations using array comparative genomic hybridization. *Curr Genomics.* 2012;13:463–70.

102. McCoy RC et al. Evidence of selection against complex mitotic-origin aneuploidy during preimplantation development. *PLOS Genet.* 2015;11:e1005601.

103. Penrose LS. The relative effects of paternal and maternal age in mongolism. 1933. *J Genet.* 2009; 88:9–14.

104. Rubio C et al. Clinical application of embryo aneuploidy testing by next-generation sequencing. *Biol Reprod.* 2019;101(6):1083–90.

105. Tarin JJ, Vendrell FJ, Ten J, Blanes R, van Blerkom J, Cano A. The oxidizing agent tertiary butyl hydroperoxide induces disturbances in spindle organization, c-meiosis, and aneuploidy in mouse oocytes. *Mol Hum Reprod.* 1996;2:895–901.

106. Tatone C et al. Evidence that carbonyl stress by methylglyoxal exposure induces DNA damage and spindle aberrations, affects mitochondrial integrity in mammalian oocytes and contributes to oocyte ageing. *Hum Reprod.* 2011;26:1843–59.

107. Battaglia DE, Goodwin P, Klein NA, Soules MR. Influence of maternal age on meiotic spindle assembly in oocytes from naturally cycling women. *Hum Reprod.* 1996;11:2217–22.

108. Munne S et al. Wide range of chromosome abnormalities in the embryos of young egg donors. *Reprod Biomed Online.* 2006;12:340–6.

109. Vickers AD. Delayed fertilization and chromosomal anomalies in mouse embryos. *J Reprod Fertil.* 1969;20:69–76.

110. Babariya D, Fragouli E, Alfarawati S, Spath K, Wells D. The incidence and origin of segmental aneuploidy in human oocytes and preimplantation embryos. *Hum Reprod.* 2017;32:2549–60.

111. Vera-Rodriguez M et al. Distribution patterns of segmental aneuploidies in human blastocysts identified by next-generation sequencing. *Fertil Steril.* 2016;105:1047–55 e2.

112. Martinez MC, Mendez C, Ferro J, Nicolas M, Serra V, Landeras J. Cytogenetic analysis of early nonviable pregnancies after assisted reproduction treatment. *Fertil Steril.* 2010;93:289–92.

113. Wellesley D et al. Rare chromosome abnormalities, prevalence and prenatal diagnosis rates from population-based congenital anomaly registers in Europe. *Eur J Hum Genet.* 2012;20:521–6.

114. Munne S, Weier HU, Grifo J, Cohen J. Chromosome mosaicism in human embryos. *Biol Reprod.* 1994;51:373–9.

115. Taylor TH, Gitlin SA, Patrick JL, Crain JL, Wilson JM, Griffin DK. The origin, mechanisms, incidence and clinical consequences of chromosomal mosaicism in humans. *Hum Reprod Update.* 2014;20:571–81.

116. Vazquez-Diez C, FitzHarris G. Causes and consequences of chromosome segregation error in preimplantation embryos. *Reproduction.* 2018;155:R63–76.

117. Kort DH et al. Human embryos commonly form abnormal nuclei during development: A mechanism of DNA damage, embryonic aneuploidy, and developmental arrest. *Hum Reprod.* 2016;31:312–23.
118. Capalbo A, Wright G, Elliott T, Ubaldi FM, Rienzi L, Nagy ZP. FISH reanalysis of inner cell mass and trophectoderm samples of previously array-CGH screened blastocysts shows high accuracy of diagnosis and no major diagnostic impact of mosaicism at the blastocyst stage. *Hum Reprod.* 2013;28:2298–307.
119. Coonen E et al. Anaphase lagging mainly explains chromosomal mosaicism in human preimplantation embryos. *Hum Reprod.* 2004;19:316–24.
120. Vazquez-Diez C, Yamagata K, Trivedi S, Haverfield J, FitzHarris G. Micronucleus formation causes perpetual unilateral chromosome inheritance in mouse embryos. *Proc Natl Acad Sci U S A.* 2016;113:626–31.
121. Robinson WP. Mechanisms leading to uniparental disomy and their clinical consequences. *BioEssays.* 2000;22:452–9.
122. Lightfoot DA, Kouznetsova A, Mahdy E, Wilbertz J, Hoog C. The fate of mosaic aneuploid embryos during mouse development. *Dev Biol.* 2006;289:384–94.
123. Yuan L, Liu JG, Hoja MR, Wilbertz J, Nordqvist K, Hoog C. Female germ cell aneuploidy and embryo death in mice lacking the meiosis-specific protein SCP3. *Science.* 2002;296:1115–8.
124. Los FJ, Van Opstal D, van den Berg C. The development of cytogenetically normal, abnormal and mosaic embryos: A theoretical model. *Hum Reprod Update.* 2004;10:79–94.
125. van Echten-Arends J et al. Chromosomal mosaicism in human preimplantation embryos: A systematic review. *Hum Reprod Update.* 2011;17:620–7.
126. Mertzanidou A et al. Microarray analysis reveals abnormal chromosomal complements in over 70% of 14 normally developing human embryos. *Hum Reprod.* 2013;28:256–64.
127. McCoy RC. Mosaicism in preimplantation human embryos: When chromosomal abnormalities are the norm. *Trends Genet.* 2017;33:448–63.
128. Rubio C et al. Preimplantation genetic screening using fluorescence in situ hybridization in patients with repetitive implantation failure and advanced maternal age: Two randomized trials. *Fertil Steril.* 2013;99:1400–7.
129. Evsikov S, Verlinsky Y. Mosaicism in the inner cell mass of human blastocysts. *Hum Reprod.* 1998;13:3151–5.
130. Sandalinas M, Sadowy S, Alikani M, Calderon G, Cohen J, Munne S. Developmental ability of chromosomally abnormal human embryos to develop to the blastocyst stage. *Hum Reprod.* 2001;16:1954–8.
131. Bolton H et al. Mouse model of chromosome mosaicism reveals lineage-specific depletion of aneuploid cells and normal developmental potential. *Nat Commun.* 2016;7:11165.
132. Ledbetter DH et al. Cytogenetic results from the U.S. Collaborative Study on CVS. *Prenat Diagn.* 1992;12:317–45.
133. Griffin DK, Millie EA, Redline RW, Hassold TJ, Zaragoza MV. Cytogenetic analysis of spontaneous abortions: Comparison of techniques and assessment of the incidence of confined placental mosaicism. *Am J Med Genet.* 1997;72:297–301.
134. Kalousek DK, Dill FJ. Chromosomal mosaicism confined to the placenta in human conceptions. *Science.* 1983;221:665–7.
135. Palermo GD, Colombero LT, Rosenwaks Z. The human sperm centrosome is responsible for normal syngamy and early embryonic development. *Rev Reprod* 1997;2:19–27.
136. Baart EB et al. Milder ovarian stimulation for in-vitro fertilization reduces aneuploidy in the human preimplantation embryo: A randomized controlled trial. *Hum Reprod.* 2007;22:980–8.
137. Capalbo A, Ubaldi FM, Rienzi L, Scott R, Treff N. Detecting mosaicism in trophectoderm biopsies: Current challenges and future possibilities. *Hum Reprod.* 2017;32:492–8.
138. Munne S et al. Detailed investigation into the cytogenetic constitution and pregnancy outcome of replacing mosaic blastocysts detected with the use of high-resolution next-generation sequencing. *Fertil Steril.* 2017;108:62–71 e8.
139. Tsuiko O et al. Karyotype of the blastocoel fluid demonstrates low concordance with both trophectoderm and inner cell mass. *Fertil Steril.* 2018;109:1127–34 e1.
140. Popovic M et al. Chromosomal mosaicism in human blastocysts: The ultimate challenge of preimplantation genetic testing? *Hum Reprod.* 2018;33:1342–54.
141. Cram DS et al. PGDIS Position Statement on the Transfer of Mosaic Embryos 2019. *Reprod Biomed Online.* 2019;39 Suppl 1:e1–4.

142. CoGEN. CoGEN Position Statement on Chromosomal Mosaicism Detected in Preimplantation Blastocyst Biopsies. https://ivf-worldwide.com/cogen/general/cogen-statement.html (accessed April 29, 2020).

143. Munne S, Grifo J, Wells D. Mosaicism: "Survival of the fittest" versus "no embryo left behind". *Fertil Steril.* 2016;105:1146–9.

144. Treff NR, Franasiak JM. Detection of segmental aneuploidy and mosaicism in the human preimplantation embryo: Technical considerations and limitations. *Fertil Steril.* 2017;107:27–31.

145. Munne S et al. Clinical outcomes after the transfer of blastocysts characterized as mosaic by high resolution Next Generation Sequencing- further insights. *Eur J Med Genet.* 2019:103741.

146. Spinella F et al. Extent of chromosomal mosaicism influences the clinical outcome of in vitro fertilization treatments. *Fertil Steril.* 2018;109:77–83.

147. Greco E, Minasi MG, Fiorentino F. Healthy Babies after Intrauterine Transfer of Mosaic Aneuploid Blastocysts. *N Engl J Med.* 2015;373:2089–90.

148. Capalbo A, Rienzi L. Mosaicism between trophectoderm and inner cell mass. *Fertil Steril.* 2017;107:1098–106.

149. Victor AR et al. Assessment of aneuploidy concordance between clinical trophectoderm biopsy and blastocyst. *Hum Reprod.* 2019;34:181–92.

150. Popovic M et al. Extended *in vitro* culture of human embryos demonstrates the complex nature of diagnosing chromosomal mosaicism from a single trophectoderm biopsy. *Hum Reprod.* 2019;34:758–69.

151. Grati FR et al. Outcomes in pregnancies with a confined placental mosaicism and implications for prenatal screening using cell-free DNA. *Genet Med.* 2019.

152. Harton GL, Cinnioglu C, Fiorentino F. Current experience concerning mosaic embryos diagnosed during preimplantation genetic screening. *Fertil Steril.* 2017;107:1113–9.

153. Diez-Juan A et al. Mitochondrial DNA content as a viability score in human euploid embryos: Less is better. *Fertil Steril.* 2015;104:534–41 e1.

154. Fragouli E et al. Altered levels of mitochondrial DNA are associated with female age, aneuploidy, and provide an independent measure of embryonic implantation potential. *PLoS Genet.* 2015;11:e1005241.

155. Fragouli E et al. Clinical implications of mitochondrial DNA quantification on pregnancy outcomes: A blinded prospective non-selection study. *Hum Reprod.* 2017;32:2340–7.

156. Ravichandran K et al. Mitochondrial DNA quantification as a tool for embryo viability assessment: Retrospective analysis of data from single euploid blastocyst transfers. *Hum Reprod.* 2017;32:1282–92.

157. Klimczak AM et al. Embryonal mitochondrial DNA: Relationship to embryo quality and transfer outcomes. *J Assist Reprod Genet.* 2018;35:871–7.

158. Shang W et al. Comprehensive chromosomal and mitochondrial copy number profiling in human IVF embryos. *Reprod Biomed Online.* 2018;36:67–74.

159. Treff NR et al. Levels of trophectoderm mitochondrial DNA do not predict the reproductive potential of sibling embryos. *Hum Reprod.* 2017;32:954–62.

160. Victor AR et al. Accurate quantitation of mitochondrial DNA reveals uniform levels in human blastocysts irrespective of ploidy, age, or implantation potential. *Fertil Steril.* 2017;107:34–42 e3.

161. Wells D. Mitochondrial DNA quantity as a biomarker for blastocyst implantation potential. *Fertil Steril.* 2017;108:742–7.

162. Victor A et al. Births from embryos with highly elevated levels of mitochondrial DNA. *Reprod Biomed Online.* 2019;39:403–12.

163. Jensen PL et al. Proteomic analysis of human blastocoel fluid and blastocyst cells. *Stem Cells Dev.* 2013;22:1126–35.

164. Zhang Y et al. Molecular analysis of DNA in blastocoele fluid using next-generation sequencing. *J Assist Reprod Genet.* 2016;33:637–45.

165. Gianaroli L et al. Blastocentesis: A source of DNA for preimplantation genetic testing. Results from a pilot study. *Fertil Steril.* 2014;102:1692–9 e6.

166. Magli MC et al. Preimplantation genetic testing: Polar bodies, blastomeres, trophectoderm cells, or blastocoelic fluid? *Fertil Steril.* 2016;105:676–83 e5.

167. Magli MC, Albanese C, Crippa A, Tabanelli C, Ferraretti AP, Gianaroli L. Deoxyribonucleic acid detection in blastocoelic fluid: A new predictor of embryo ploidy and viable pregnancy. *Fertil Steril.* 2019;111:77–85.

168. Brison DR et al. Identification of viable embryos in IVF by non-invasive measurement of amino acid turnover. *Hum Reprod.* 2004;19:2319–24.

169. Houghton FD et al. Non-invasive amino acid turnover predicts human embryo developmental capacity. *Hum Reprod.* 2002;17:999–1005.

170. Huang L, Bogale B, Tang Y, Lu S, Xie XS, Racowsky C. Noninvasive preimplantation genetic testing for aneuploidy in spent medium may be more reliable than trophectoderm biopsy. *Proc Natl Acad Sci U S A.* 2019;116:14105–12.

171. Jiao J et al. Minimally invasive preimplantation genetic testing using blastocyst culture medium. *Hum Reprod.* 2019;34:1369–79.

172. Kuznyetsov V et al. Evaluation of a novel non-invasive preimplantation genetic screening approach. *PLOS ONE* 2018;13:e0197262.

173. Li P et al. Preimplantation genetic screening with spent culture medium/blastocoel fluid for in vitro fertilization. *Sci Rep.* 2018;8:9275.

174. Xu J et al. Noninvasive chromosome screening of human embryos by genome sequencing of embryo culture medium for in vitro fertilization. *Proc Natl Acad Sci U S A.* 2016;113:11907–12.

175. Rubio C et al. Embryonic cell-free DNA versus trophectoderm biopsy for aneuploidy testing: Concordance rate and clinical implications. *Fertil Steril.* 2019;112:510–9.

176. Ferreux L et al. Live birth rate following frozen-thawed blastocyst transfer is higher with blastocysts expanded on Day 5 than on Day 6. *Hum Reprod.* 2018;33:390–8.

177. Vera-Rodriguez M et al. Origin and composition of cell-free DNA in spent medium from human embryo culture during preimplantation development. *Hum Reprod.* 2018;33:745–56.

178. Basile N et al. Increasing the probability of selecting chromosomally normal embryos by time-lapse morphokinetics analysis. *Fertil Steril.* 2014;101:699–704.

179. Campbell A, Fishel S, Bowman N, Duffy S, Sedler M, Hickman CF. Modelling a risk classification of aneuploidy in human embryos using non-invasive morphokinetics. *Reprod Biomed Online.* 2013;26:477–85.

180. Chavez SL et al. Dynamic blastomere behaviour reflects human embryo ploidy by the four-cell stage. *Nat Commun.* 2012;3:1251.

181. Del Carmen Nogales M et al. Type of chromosome abnormality affects embryo morphology dynamics. *Fertil Steril.* 2017;107:229–35 e2.

182. Yang Z et al. Selection of competent blastocysts for transfer by combining time-lapse monitoring and array CGH testing for patients undergoing preimplantation genetic screening: A prospective study with sibling oocytes. *BMC Med Genomics* 2014;7:38.

183. Patel DV, Shah PB, Kotdawala AP, Herrero J, Rubio I, Banker MR. Morphokinetic behavior of euploid and aneuploid embryos analyzed by time-lapse in embryoscope. *J Hum Reprod Sci* 2016;9:112–8.

184. Reignier A, Lammers J, Barriere P, Freour T. Can time-lapse parameters predict embryo ploidy? A systematic review. *Reprod Biomed Online.* 2018;36:380–7.

185. Meseguer M, Herrero J, Tejera A, Hilligsoe KM, Ramsing NB, Remohi J. The use of morphokinetics as a predictor of embryo implantation. *Hum Reprod.* 2011;26:2658–71.

186. Campbell A, Fishel S, Bowman N, Duffy S, Sedler M, Thornton S. Retrospective analysis of outcomes after IVF using an aneuploidy risk model derived from time-lapse imaging without PGS. *Reprod Biomed Online.* 2013;27:140–6.

187. Mumusoglu S et al. Duration of blastulation may be associated with ongoing pregnancy rate in single euploid blastocyst transfer cycles. *Reprod Biomed Online.* 2017;35:633–9.

4

Preimplantation Genetic Testing for Structural Rearrangements

Cagri Ogur and Darren K. Griffin

CONTENTS

Introduction

Structural chromosomal rearrangements (SRs) are among the major abnormalities accounting for genetic disorders and infertility [1]. Unlike aneuploidy, which is defined by copy number changes of whole chromosome(s), SRs involve abnormalities of chromosomal segments. SRs can be either balanced or unbalanced. Balanced rearrangements have no apparent overall loss or gain in genetic material and therefore carriers are often not phenotypically affected, provided that the rearrangement doesn't disrupt any key functional genes. They are, however, at increased risk of infertility, miscarriage, stillbirth, and liveborns with mental and/or physical disabilities due to increased risk of producing chromosomally unbalanced gametes [2]. Male carriers often have altered semen parameters and fertility problems such that the incidence of translocations is 6.5- to 9.4-fold higher in infertile males than in newborn population [3]. The reproductive risk of a carrier couple is affected by factors such as the type of SR, the chromosomes involved, the breakpoints, segregational tendencies, family history, female age, sperm parameters, and ovarian reserve [4].

In order to minimize the risks associated with SRs, prenatal and preimplantation genetic testing are the two interventions currently offered to carrier couples. Prenatal testing, however, involves the analysis of an already established pregnancy, and the couple might have to experience the burden of termination if the fetus is diagnosed as "unbalanced." Moreover, without the help of assisted reproductive techniques, carrier couples might have to wait longer periods to achieve an implantation and a clinically recognized pregnancy, depending on their aforementioned reproductive risks. Preimplantation genetic testing-structural chromosome rearrangements (PGT-SR) offers a unique opportunity to maximize the chances of a successful implantation and minimize the risks of reproductive wastage with the selection and the transfer of only normal or balanced (normal/balanced) embryos [5]. Since the 1990s, PGT-SR has been a frequent indication in the context of IVF and the number is growing yearly, with more carrier patients being identified. According to the multicenter analysis from the European Society of Human Reproduction and Embryology (ESHRE) consortium, 4253 cycles had been performed for structural chromosomal abnormalities within 10 years (1997–2007), with an increasing trend upward in the number of cycles with each year [6]. More contemporary world figures are harder to find; however, it is clear from personal communications from diagnostic labs that numbers are on the rise.

A variety of different genetic analysis techniques have been used in the selection of normal/balanced embryos, including fluorescence *in situ* hybridization (FISH), comparative genomic hybridization (CGH), array-CGH (aCGH), single nucleotide polymorphism (SNP)-arrays, karyomapping, and next-generation sequencing (NGS). Different biopsy strategies and sampling methods include pre- and post-conception approaches, including polar body, cleavage stage, blastocyst stage biopsy, and more recently, noninvasive testing methods (reviewed in [7] and in Chapter 3 of this book).

The aim of this chapter is to review the types of balanced rearrangements, likely outcomes, analysis techniques, applications of PGT-SR, and current clinical outcomes.

The Origin and the Types of Balanced Rearrangements

SRs are formed via double-stranded breaks and subsequent joining of those breakpoints by DNA repair machinery [8]. This creates derivative chromosomes where the order and the linkage relationships of genes differ. They can be formed in any of the chromosomes; however, there are hot-spots or frequent breakpoints in the genome. Mechanisms such as non-allelic homologous recombination (NAHR) [9,10], DNA double strand break repair via non-homologous end-joining (NHEJ) [8,11], microhomology-mediated break-induced replication (MMBIR), fork stalling and template switching (FoSTeS) [12], "chromothripsis" [1,13], palindrome-mediated mechanisms [14], nucleolar localization of chromosomes, and exposure to chemicals and radiation [15] are thought to be responsible in the generation of rearrangements. Within the scope of PGT-SR, the types and the reproductive outcomes of rearrangement carriers are usually restricted to balanced reciprocal and Robertsonian translocations (RecT and RobT), inversions, complex chromosome rearrangements, and insertions (Figure 4.1).

In most cases, SRs are found to be inherited from carrier parents, and are thus familial (Figure 4.2) [16,17]. According to a large survey based on 24,951 prenatal samples, the rate of inherited balanced rearrangements was 26–28 per 10,000 fetuses, whereas *de novo* balanced abnormalities were 7.6–9.6 per 10,000 [16]. The same rearrangement can result in different reproductive risks in different carriers (even siblings) depending on the sex, age, gonadal reserve, and other clinical characteristics. Thus, genetic counseling in the light of proper family history is vital in order to make a risk assessment. *De novo* SRs arise by the aforementioned mechanisms during gametogenesis [16]. Should the rearrangement be formed in the germline, it might be inherited through generations with no apparent previous history in the family. For example, the t(11;22) translocation in all its *de novo* forms is of paternal origin, suggesting a sperm-specific mechanism of t(11;22) formation [18].

Reciprocal Translocations

Reciprocal translocations (RecT) occur by an exchange of segments between two non-homologous chromosomes, producing two derivatives (der), which are named according to their centromeres

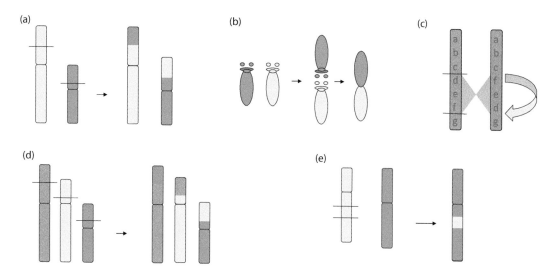

FIGURE 4.1 (a) Balanced reciprocal translocation (RecT) between nonhomologous chromosomes. (b) Robertsonian translocation (RobT) between two acrocentric chromosomes. (c) Paracentric inversion on q arm. (d) Complex chromosomal rearrangement involving three chromosomes. (e) Insertional translocation by the insertion of a chromosomal segment into another chromosome.

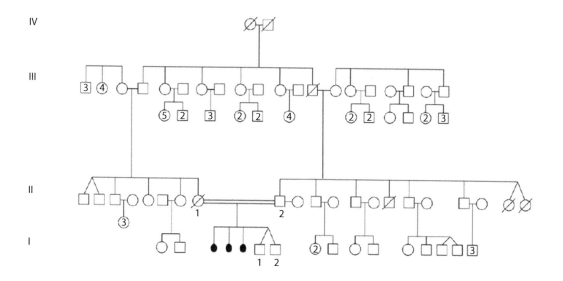

FIGURE 4.2 A complex pedigree where the translocation was inherited through at least three generations. In that case, the reproductive outcome got worse after the last generation made a consanguineous marriage with both partners (II.1 and II.2) carrying the same reciprocal translocation. The numbers inside the circles and squares indicate the number of children born with the same gender. (From Beyazyurek C et al. *Fertil Steril.* 1 May, 2010;93(7):2413.e1–5. With permission.)

(Figure 4.1a). They are among the most common structural abnormalities, with an estimated incidence of 1 in 600 live births [19], and 5.7% among couples with recurrent miscarriages [2]. Balanced RecT are copy-number neutral; therefore, carriers have a normal phenotype. However, they have a high risk of producing chromosomally unbalanced gametes through abnormal segregations.

Homologous pairing and recombination play a critical role in meiosis. In a normal individual, during the pachytene stage of meiosis I, each chromosome pairs with its homolog and they are held together until they are segregated properly to the poles at the end of anaphase. However, in RecT carriers, in order to allow homologous synapsis to occur, the four chromosomes (two derivatives and two normal homologs) form a "quadrivalent" (Figure 4.3). During anaphase I, there are five major possibilities for segregation of those chromosomes: alternate, adjacent-1, adjacent-2, 3:1, and 4:0 (Figure 4.4). With the addition of the recombination events within the segments resulting in asymmetric segregation in meiosis II and meiotic non-disjunctions in anaphase II, up to 32 different gametes could be produced, of which only 2 arising from alternate segregation could give rise to normal/balanced embryos (Table 4.1) (reviewed in [20]).

During alternate segregation, the two normal chromosomes (termed A and B) and two derivatives (derA and derB) segregate to the opposite poles producing either normal or carrier gametes, respectively. In adjacent-1 segregation, the two adjacent chromosomes with homologous centromeres segregate to the opposite poles. Resulting embryos would have partial monosomy/partial trisomy of the translocated segments, respectively. This is the most frequent segregation mode found in the zygotes and could be associated with viable imbalances. In adjacent-2 segregation, the two adjacent chromosomes with homologous centromeres segregate to the same pole. The resulting embryo would have partial monosomy/trisomy of the centric segments, which often result in non-viable embryos. In 3:1 segregation mode, any of the three chromosomes segregate together to the same pole, and one remaining segregates to the opposite pole. This mode leads to tertiary and interchange trisomy/monosomy of the chromosomes. Finally, 4:0 segregation results in double monosomy or double trisomy of the chromosomes which are mostly not compatible with life (Figure 4.4) [21].

Due to the relative inaccessibility and low abundance of oocytes, the vast majority of the research on segregation patterns comes from the assessment of spermatozoa. Sperm karyotyping using the technique of human sperm–hamster oocyte fusion was the first method used for analysis [22]. Although this technique provides a direct investigation and a comprehensive view of all numerical and structural chromosomal abnormalities, it is time consuming and the yield is low. Later, it was replaced by FISH analysis using chromosomal-specific probes, which is a faster and less laborious method that allows the analysis of thousands of sperm in one assay [23]. However, this technique is limited to the number of chromosomes analyzed due to the limited availability of probes and the filters used in imaging systems. Other limitations include difficulties in evaluation of the signals. Recently, single-sperm analysis by aCGH seemed to overcome the disadvantages of both former methods [24]. In one study, 43 sperm from a man with a balanced translocation [46,XY,t(2;12)(p11.2;q24.31)] were analyzed by aCGH, which showed gains and losses corresponding to the regions involved in the translocation in 18.6% and alterations in other chromosomes in 16.3% of sperm [24]. Studies, however, show considerable heterogeneity in both the percentage of unbalanced sperm and the segregational characteristics. Based on the analysis of 136 reciprocal translocation heterozygotes, unbalanced spermatozoa were detected in male carriers of balanced reciprocal translocations with a frequency of 19%–91% (reviewed in [25]).

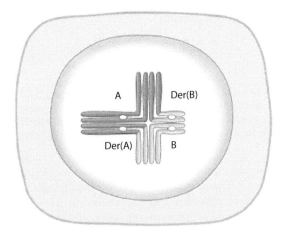

FIGURE 4.3   Quadrivalent structure arising at meiosis from a RecT. Chromosomes A, B, Der(A), and Der(B) are indicated.

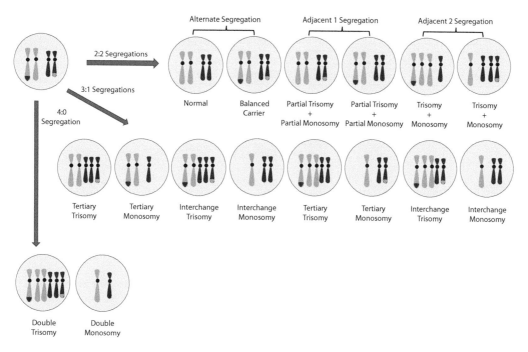

FIGURE 4.4 Segregation modes of a reciprocal translocation. The resulting embryos are shown assuming the other partner contributes normal chromosomes [21] (only major segregation modes are shown for simplicity). *2:2 Alternate segregation:* Two normal chromosomes and two derivatives segregate to the opposite poles producing either normal or balanced gametes, respectively. *2:2 Adjacent-1:* Two adjacent chromosomes with homologous centromeres segregate to the opposite poles. Resulting embryos would have partial monosomy/partial trisomy of the translocated segments, respectively. *2:2 Adjacent-2:* Two adjacent chromosomes with homologous centromeres segregate to the same pole. Resulting embryo would have partial monosomy/trisomy of the centric segments. *3:1 segregation:* Three chromosomes segregate to the same pole and one chromosome segregates to the opposite pole. This mode leads to tertiary and interchange trisomy/monosomy of the chromosomes. *4:0 segregation:* This mode leads to double monosomy or double trisomy of the chromosomes where all chromosomes are pulled to one pole leaving null to the other. (Adapted from Beyer CE et al. *J Assist Reprod Genet.* Nov 2017;34(11):1483–92.)

Recombination within the homologous regions of the interstitial segments is another factor that decreases the proportion of balanced/normal gametes [26]. The frequency of recombination depends on the length of the segments and the efficiency of the synapsis established between the chromosomes. Although segment size and the presence of heterochromatin regions play important roles, recombination behavior within a quadrivalent of a given chromosome is not predictable. The same chromosome can display different chiasmata distributions depending on the translocation and the segment size. Therefore, each carrier has a unique risk associated with their rearrangement and reproductive outcome. In the context of PGT-SR, patients need to be properly genetically counseled as to the range of outcomes that could arise as a result of their balanced rearrangement.

Although the frequencies of segregation types observed in sperm and embryos may not have a one-to-one correlation due to some postzygotic selection against some of the unbalanced genotypes, a strong correlation has been found between the percentage of abnormal gametes and the percentage of abnormal embryos in RecT carriers [27]. This demonstrates that the proportion of unbalanced spermatozoa in reciprocal translocation carriers could serve as a predictive value on embryonic outcomes in PGT-SR treatments; however, if the female partner is the carrier, risk cannot so easily be assessed prior to PGT-SR.

TABLE 4.1

Possible Segregation Modes of a Reciprocal Translocation between A and B Seen in Figure 4.1[a]

Segregation Mode	Segregational Products/Gametes	Chromosome Composition in Zygote	Result
2:2 alternate	A,B	A,A,B,B	Normal
	der(A),der(B)	A,der(A),B,der(B)	Balanced
2:2 adjacent-I	A,der(B)	A,A,B,der(B)	Partial trisomy (TS-A), partial monosomy (TS of B)
	B,der(A)	A,der(A),B,B	Partial monosomy (TS of A), partial trisomy (TS of B)
2:2 adjacent-II	A,der(A)	A,A,der(A),B	Partial trisomy (CS of A), partial monosomy (CS of B)
	B,der(B)	A,B,der(B)	Partial monosomy (CS of A), partial trisomy (CS of B)
3:1	A	A,A,B	Interchange monosomy (B)
	B,der(A),der(B)	A,der(A),B,B,der(B)	Interchange trisomy (B)
	B	A,B,B	Interchange monosomy (A)
	A,der(A),der(B)	A,A,der(A),B,der(B)	Interchange trisomy (A)
	der(A)	A,der(A),B	Tertiary monosomy (TS of A), tertiary monosomy (CS of B)
	A,B,der(B)	A,A,B,B,der(B)	Tertiary trisomy (TS of A), tertiary trisomy (CS of B)
	der(B)	A,B,der(B)	Tertiary monosomy (CS of A), tertiary monosomy (TS of B)
	A,B,der(A)	A,A,B,B,der(A)	Tertiary trisomy (CS of A), tertiary trisomy (TS of B)
4:0	A,B,der(A),der(B)	A,A,B,B,der(A),der(B)	Double trisomy (A and B)
	NULL	A,B	Double monosomy (A and B)

Abbreviations: TS, translocated segment; CS, centric segment.
[a] Non-disjunction and crossing over events were disregarded for simplicity.

Robertsonian Translocations

Robertsonian translocations (RobT) result from breakage of two acrocentric chromosomes (13, 14, 15, 21, and 22) and subsequent fusion of their long arms to form one derivative chromosome (Figure 4.1b). The short arms are lost, and the total chromosome number is reduced to 45. Since short arms have only repetitive sequences coding nucleolar organizer (NOR) genes, their absence is not associated with any phenotypic consequences. The incidence of RobT is 1 in 1085 births [3]. During meiosis I, derivative and normal chromosomes pair as a "trivalent." There are three segregation modes: alternate, adjacent, and 3:0. In alternate segregation, the derivative chromosome segregates into one pole and both normal chromosomes segregate to the other pole, producing a carrier or a normal gamete, respectively. In adjacent segregation, the derivative chromosome segregates together with one of the normal chromosomes, and the other normal chromosome segregates to the other pole producing either disomic and/or nullisomic gametes, leading to trisomic/monosomic embryos. The 3:0 segregation is very rare and produces double disomy/nullisomy in gametes and double trisomy/monosomy in embryos (Figure 4.5). Sperm karyotyping and FISH studies demonstrate that the frequency of abnormal gametes ranges from 3% to 40% (reviewed [25]). The natural tendency of the trivalent having a cis configuration [28] might have an influence on the high rate of normal/balanced gametes via increasing the probability of alternate segregation.

Inversions

Inversions occur after two double-strand breaks are formed on the same chromosome followed by 180° rotation of the segment before reunion. In balanced inversions, there is no loss or gain in genetic material; however, the gene order is changed. There are two types of inversions, categorized by the position of the

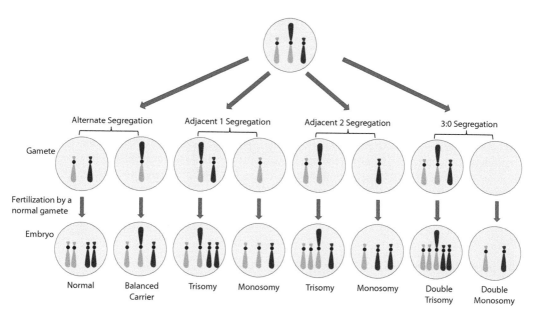

FIGURE 4.5 Segregation modes of Robertsonian translocation. (Adapted from Beyer CE et al. *J Assist Reprod Genet.* Nov 2017;34(11):1483–92.)

centromere. Paracentric inversions (PAI) occur when both breakpoints are in the same chromosome arm (Figure 4.1c), whereas pericentric inversions (PEI) occur when the breakpoints are in different arms and the inverted segment involves the centromere. The incidence of PAI is estimated to be 0.1%–0.5% [29]. There are serious reproductive risks associated with inversions depending on the chromosomes involved, the size, and the distribution of the euchromatic regions within the inverted segment. During pachytene, an inversion loop might form in order to have a homologous synapse between the inverted and non-inverted regions. In PAI carriers, if an odd number of crossovers occur within the loop, acentric fragments (which are lost) and dicentric bridges are formed that will eventually be split up and produce unbalanced gametes (Figure 4.6). In PEI carriers, the outcome is partial duplication/deletion of the distal parts of the inversion, resulting in an embryo with partial monosomy and partial trisomy [30]. PAI are rare and are generally considered harmless due to their low risk of production of unbalanced gametes. The rate of recombinant sperm ranges from 0% to 12.6% [31,32]. The low risk observed in those studies suggests, for most of the inversions, either an inversion loop is not formed, or crossing over is suppressed during meiosis. However, more recently, Yapan and colleagues showed that a high proportion of unbalanced gametes (28%) might also be formed in the case of large paracentric inversions, demonstrating that the reproductive risks are associated mostly to the segment size, which increases the likelihood of recombination events within the inverted segment [33].

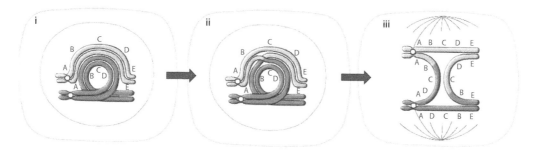

FIGURE 4.6 Loop formation in a PAI carrier (i); after crossing-over event (ii); dicentric bridge and acentric fragment are formed (iii).

The frequency of unbalanced spermatozoa from inversion carriers varies from 0% to 54% (reviewed [25]). Morel and colleagues found a significant correlation between the relative size of the inversion and the frequency of recombination ($R = 0.76$, $p = 0.001$). No recombinant chromosomes were produced when the inverted segment involved <30% of the chromosome length (independent of the size of the inverted segment) [34].

The most commonly reported inversion is a PEI of chromosome 9, specifically inv(9)(p11q12) and inv(9)(p11q13), thought to occur in 0.25%–3.5%, depending on the population studied [35]. The clinical significance is not entirely clear, and some reports are conflicting (with many suggesting it is a normal variant) but it has been associated with infertility, recurrent pregnancy loss, cancer, congenital anomalies, and growth retardation [36]. Its relatively high frequency is thought to be due to its structural organization involving the pericentric region just below the centromere, making it more prone to breakage. In summary, the genetic risk of inversions is mostly related to the chromosome involved, the proportion of the segment that is inverted, and the incidence of recombination within the segment [33,34,37]. In the context of counseling for PGT-SR, all these factors need to be taken into account.

Complex Chromosomal Rearrangements

Complex chromosomal rearrangements (CCR) are defined as structural rearrangements mostly formed by (i) two separate simple rearrangements in the same individual (double translocation), (ii) terminal exchanges involving three chromosomes with one breakpoint in each chromosome (three-way translocation), and (iii) more complex rearrangements with multiple breakpoints involving more than three chromosomes (Figure 4.1d) [38]. They are extremely rare in the population, and the majority of CCR (~70%) are *de novo* in origin [147]. In the case of three-way complex translocations, hexavalent configurations are expected to be formed during meiosis [38,147], which decreases the chances of balanced gamete formation and identifying normal/balanced embryos. In a retrospective analysis of PGT-SR for seven carriers with CCR, only 5.9% of the embryos were found to be normal/balanced [148]. These are perhaps the most difficult to counsel for in the context of PGT-SR.

Insertional Translocations

Balanced insertional translocations constitute an important part of complex chromosomal rearrangements. They occur by the intercalation of a part of one chromosome into another non-homologous chromosome (interchromosomal) (Figure 4.1e) or into another part of the same chromosome (intrachromosomal). They are difficult to identify with classical cytogenetic techniques and occur very rarely, with an incidence of less than 1 in 1300 [126]. Sperm FISH using locus-specific probes might be a good predictor to assess the risk of male carriers and to inform the patient with better genetic counseling [39]. Since this type of translocation is very rare and because of the lack of availability of locus-specific probes for each chromosomal region, there is only limited experience and data on the success and availability of PGT-SR on insertional translocations [40,41]. However, with the advancement of comprehensive methods such as aCGH and NGS, preparation of specific probes is no longer needed [42]. Jones and colleagues performed the first PGT-SR for a carrier of intrachromosomal insertion using aCGH [137]. The analysis of six blastocysts revealed that 67% of the embryos were unbalanced. Unfortunately, no pregnancy was achieved after the transfer of two normal/balanced embryos in this case [137].

PGT-SR in Practice

PGT-SR is routinely offered to patients carrying balanced rearrangements with a view to reducing the risk of IVF failure, miscarriage, or congenital birth defects. A variety of different genetic analysis techniques have been used so far in the selection of normal/balanced embryos, including FISH, array-based techniques, and NGS, coupled with different biopsy strategies and sampling methods. These largely mirror those used for PGT-A.

Sampling Methods

There are currently both invasive and noninvasive screening methods for PGT-SR. Invasive methods include polar body (PB1 and PB2), cleavage-stage (blastomere), and blastocyst-stage (trophectoderm tissue) biopsies ([7] and in Chapter 3 of this book). There are both advantages and disadvantages of each technique in the context of PGT-SR. Pre-conceptional diagnosis (polar body biopsy) is performed before fertilization and is being used only for maternally transmitted rearrangements as a means of PGT-SR in countries where PGT in embryos is restricted [43,44]. Cleavage-stage and blastocyst biopsy proceed as for all forms of PGT, with blastocyst now becoming the most common, as it has been shown to have no negative effect, while cleavage-stage biopsy reduces implantation rates significantly [45].

Recent studies have shown that blastocoel fluid and spent blastocyst medium could potentially serve as alternative sources for template DNA sampling for the diagnosis of both numerical and segmental aneuploidy of the early embryo [46–48]. For blastocoel fluid sampling alone, the concordance rate between the diagnosis results of trophectoderm samples from the same embryo is high (97.1%). The amplification rate (82%) is not ideal, however, and it may still require an invasive biopsy for a significant proportion of the embryos to have a confirmatory diagnosis of the segregational status of the chromosomes [47]. Assessment of spent culture medium sampling for PGT-SR has been successfully applied on a patient with a male carrier of a balanced translocation [46,XY,t(14;15)(q22;q24)] which resulted in the live birth of a chromosomally normal and a healthy baby [49]. Recently, a combination of both blastocoel fluid and spent culture medium made an improvement in the accuracy of the diagnosis. Jiao et al. [50] first systematically performed PGT-SR on mixed blastocoel fluid and spent blastocyst medium, trophectoderm (TE), and whole embryo samples while making significant modifications to the pre-existing multiple annealing and looping-based amplification cycle (MALBAC) techniques used for DNA amplification [50]. Using this combination, 41 blastocysts donated by 22 couples known to carry a chromosome rearrangement were successfully quantified by segmental abnormalities with high resolution ($\sim$1 Mb), and in none of the samples was maternal contamination detected [50].

FISH

Fluorescence *in situ* hybridization (FISH) is one of the oldest methods used in the diagnosis of chromosomal abnormalities, but on the whole, less controversial in the context of PGT-SR than PGT-A. Unlike the non-targeted PGT-A, FISH-based PGT-SR involves the identification of specific loci (typically centromeres and subtelomeric regions) with fluorescently labeled probes that are complementary to the specific DNA regions. First introduced into IVF in 1991 by using X- and Y-chromosomal specific probes in order to select disease-free embryos for X-linked disorders [51], this method was also used later in the diagnosis of aneuploidy [52] and then unbalanced products of rearrangement carriers [53]. The approaches mostly involved using locus-specific probes in interphase cells and a three-color strategy (either one centromeric and two subtelomeric or two centromeric and one subtelomeric probe), which has been used routinely to detect nearly all segregational abnormalities [54,55].

One of the biggest limitations of this approach, however, is the need for pre-clinical workup in order to confirm the breakpoints and signal specificities, which may involve analysis of at least 10 metaphase cells and 100 interphase cells on each carrier's peripheral blood sample. This is time consuming and thus costly. Fixation is another limiting step in obtaining good-quality nucleus, which is highly dependent on the technical skills of the performer. There are three main fixation methods [56], where the most routinely used protocol involves hypotonic solution and Carnoy's fixative (3:1 methanol-acetic acid). An inappropriate fixation might cause losing of nuclear material and/or poor hybridization. Depending on the probes and the success of the fixation, artifacts and non-specific signals might cause diagnostic errors.

The availability of different fluorochrome probes specific for the chromosomal regions is another limitation. Moreover, the fact that a significant proportion of aneuploidies seen in PGT-SR cases are not related to the translocation [57], a significant number of aneuploidies are not assayed and thus the approach has largely been replaced by comprehensive chromosomal screening techniques. However, FISH still has a place in the case of cryptic translocations and inversions, since most of the comprehensive chromosome screening methods are not able to give reliable results for small rearrangements less than 2 Mb.

Until comprehensive chromosomal analysis techniques such as aCGH and NGS systems came along, researchers tried to improve the informativity of the FISH system both quantitively (adding extra probes for aneuploidy) and qualitatively, such that it could also distinguish a balanced chromosome complement from a normal one. For this reason, carrier-specific probes were developed to be used in interphase cells [53]. This approach was based on hybridization of breakpoint spanning yeast artificial chromosome (YAC) DNA probes; however, it requires a major pre-clinical work up developing those probes for each specific translocation.

Another approach within FISH-based PGT-SR for distinguishing normal embryos from carriers was using FISH on metaphase chromosomes from single blastomeres using conversion via nuclear transfer or chemical solutions [58,59]. In order to create metaphase preparations, single blastomeres were fused with enucleated or intact mouse zygotes (nuclear transfer) or were treated with caffeine and colcemid [59]. The nuclear transfer technique was applied to 437 blastomeres, of which 88% resulted in successful nuclear conversion and a 29% of clinical pregnancy rate per transfer, with 7 healthy deliveries in 52 cycles [58]. In a larger study, including the results of the previous experience, a chemical conversion method was applied to 946 blastomeres in 94 cycles with 71% efficiency, leading to a conversion rate that decreased spontaneous abortion to 13%–15%, compared to their PB1/PB2 control group (25%) [59]. Nevertheless, this technique is labor-intensive and limited by the availability of fertilized mouse zygotes and the efficiency of the conversion method.

Most of the PGT-SR with FISH was performed without additional aneuploidy screening [60,61], and thus only a few have yielded results of chromosomal abnormalities unrelated to translocations [62–64]. The rate of abnormalities not involved in translocations has been found to be relatively frequent in embryos obtained from RobT carriers, which were higher than RecT carriers (67% vs. 22%) [62]. In another study, an overall 60.3% aneuploidy rate was found after the analysis of five chromosomes (13, 16, 18, 21, 22) in cleavage-stage embryos of 13 RecT carriers [63]. Only 8.7% of them were both normal/balanced and euploid for the five chromosomes, thus transferable. Here, the aneuploidy rate was similar when compared between sexes and between age groups ($\leq$37 and >37 years old) but differed among normal/balanced embryos and unbalanced embryos. Aneuploid embryos were more likely to have unbalanced complement, suggesting a global disruption of mitotic and meiotic segregations of chromosomes. Embryo transfer was performed for nine carriers but unfortunately no clinical pregnancy was achieved in this cohort. In another study where aneuploidy screening was performed in RecT carriers for chromosomes 13, 18, 21, X, and Y revealed that 46.8% of 141 embryos were aneuploid. The live birth rate was 26.7% per embryo transfer; however, the authors concluded that additional aneuploidy screening did not improve the clinical outcomes [64].

The reproductive history of rearrangement carrier couples before PGT-SR treatment is mostly unsuccessful, with live-born delivery rates of around 4.8%–9.7% [64]. Several studies claimed that they observed an increase in live birth rate and decrease in miscarriage rate after PGT-SR compared to natural conception and cycles without PGT-SR. Munne and colleagues performed PGT-SR for 35 cases that demonstrated statistically significant decreases in spontaneous abortions from 92% of the pregnancies in natural conceptions to 12.5% in PGD cycles (p < 0.001) [54]. In another study, after PGT-SR, 24.7% implantation rate and 18.6% miscarriage rate were obtained, and take-home baby rate was increased from 11.5% to 81.4% per pregnancy achieved [65]. In another study population, PGT-SR was able to dramatically increase the live birth rate up to 85.7% once there was a positive β-hCG [64].

Whatever attempts have been made to make FISH a better diagnostic technique, it failed to improve live birth rates consistently, possibly due to additional drawbacks of cleavage-stage biopsy [45], which was predominantly used at that time period (before 2010). According to the ESHRE PGD consortium data, the clinical pregnancy rate was 12%–17% per oocyte retrieved and 22%–26% per embryo transferred, which was not favorable [6]. In a systematic review, the reproductive outcomes of couples after PGT-SR were compared with the outcomes of natural conceptions of rearrangement carriers [66]. This study included 4 observational studies including 469 couples with natural conception and 21 studies including 126 couples undergoing PGT-SR. According to this study, the live birth rate per couple varied between 33% and 60% (median 34%) in the natural conception group, whereas after PGT-SR, it varied between 0 and 100% (median 31%). The miscarriage rate appeared to improve overall, but not significantly, which resulted in 21%–40% (median 34%) in natural conception and

0%–50% (median 0%) after PGT-SR. Unfortunately, information about the time required to obtain a healthy live birth was not present in this study since none of the included reports provided enough information on this parameter. Recently, another meta-analysis [67] demonstrated that similar live birth rate, time to conception, and miscarriage rates are observed through natural conception and PGT-SR in couples with structural abnormality and experiencing recurrent pregnancy loss. The time frame of this analysis includes 1997–2014, which obviously highlights the heterogeneity of the studies including clinical characteristics of patients and the techniques used. In addition, these reviews were limited only to couples who have at least two or more miscarriages and thus lacks the results of translocation carriers who are diagnosed with primary infertility. A significant proportion of rearrangement carriers fail to conceive due to patient-specific factors and some additional male factor involvement, which together make the use of assisted reproduction techniques and intracytoplasmic sperm injection (ICSI) technique as an obligatory choice.

STR Typing

Short-tandem repeat (STR) typing involves the application of a PCR-based protocol using multiplexed STR markers located on both sides of the breakpoint [68]. An extensive workup is required specific to the translocation in question. A total of 29 patients were analyzed by this method and the proportion of alternate segregation for RecT and RobT was 33% and 77%, respectively [68]. The fetal heartbeat rate was 46% for RecT and 40% for RobT carriers. This technique might also provide an additional control for contamination of exogenous DNA, detection of uniparental disomy (UPD), and the possibility of adding extra markers for aneuploidy for other chromosomes [69]. In another study, a total 241 embryos were analyzed from 27 couples using a similar multiplex STR system. In this cohort, the frequency of alternate segregations was 38.5% and 66.1% for RecT and RobT carriers, respectively. A total of 90 embryos were also tested for aneuploidy for 9 other chromosomes (13, 14, 15, 16, 18, 21, 22, X, Y) in addition to the rearrangement, which showed that 63.1% of them were aneuploid. A relatively high rate of implantation (59.6%) was achieved possibly due to additional aneuploidy testing on the normal/balanced embryos [69]. Although these studies demonstrate the reliability of the approach, there are drawbacks in the time and cost of that workup.

CGH and aCGH

Eventually, FISH and STR-typing were replaced by comprehensive cytogenetic techniques such as aCGH and SNP-arrays. It thus became possible for the first time to detect aneuploidy and segmental imbalances simultaneously in a single biopsy material from an embryo [70,71]. The first technique that was developed for comprehensive analysis of embryos was comparative genomic hybridization (CGH), first introduced in molecular cytogenetics in 1992 to detect somatic mutations in cancer cells [72]. When applied to biopsied embryo cells, samples were amplified by whole-genome amplification (WGA) followed by co-hybridization of differentially labeled test and reference DNA on to normal metaphase chromosomes where analysis takes place on the microscope [73]. However, the resolution of this technique proved to be low (10–25 Mb) [70,74]; it is also laborious and time consuming. Malmgren et al. in 2002 analyzed 94 blastomeres from 7 couples carrying structural chromosome rearrangements, and the results were rechecked using FISH [70]. The confirmation rate between CGH and FISH was not satisfactory, possibly due to a high degree of mosaicism (~100%) and the presence of chaotic complements in the cleavage-stage embryos.

The chromosomally-based CGH technique was replaced by aCGH, which is more automated, accurate, and has a shorter protocol [75]. In this technique, instead of using metaphases, the hybridization takes place on microarrays (chips) containing thousands of bacterial artificial chromosome (BAC) clones (e.g., the 24sure+ arrays from Illumina) or with specific oligonucleotide sequences (oligo probes; Agilent Technologies). As for PGT-A, a dedicated software analyzes the ratio between the signal intensities and reports the deviations on a logarithmic scale as a gain or a loss. Depending on the platform used, BlueFuse Multi software (Illumina) for example, detects median log 2 ratio for all the chromosomes. This method cannot differentiate between normal and balanced embryos, and the resolution ranges from 5–10 Mb for

BAC arrays (although 2.5 Mb segmental imbalances were also successfully identified) [76] to 20–50 kb for oligo-arrays [77], depending on the chromosomal region and the type of chip being used. Generally speaking, this method is able to detect unbalanced embryos provided that three of the four fragments are larger than 6 Mb [78]. In a study where the diagnostic efficiencies of CGH, aCGH-BAC arrays, and aCGH-oligo arrays were compared in cleavage-stage embryos, all three techniques provided similar profiles; however, relevant to PGT-SR, the oligo-array, with its higher resolution (~20 kb), could detect extra segmental imbalances in 14.7% of the blastomeres that the other two methods had missed [77]. This approach also allowed simultaneous detection of aneuploidy and other *de novo* abnormalities unrelated to the rearrangement of the carrier parent [57,76,79,80]. In a validation study, it was found that aCGH is a more effective method than FISH, in that 26.4% of normal/balanced embryos were found to carry aneuploidy that FISH was not able to detect [79].

After a long period of FISH being the gold standard, a series of clinical studies using comprehensive chromosome screening methods, principally aCGH, demonstrated its efficacy in PGT-SR, and FISH was discontinued. The first such study [76], using cleavage-stage biopsy, achieved a 70.6% clinical pregnancy rate (CPR) and a 63.6% implantation rate (IR) per embryo transfer (ET) for a group of translocation carrier patients. The first healthy delivery was reported in a study of the same year [81] where 20 cycles were performed overall for 5 Robertsonian and 9 reciprocal translocations, plus 2 inversion carrier couples. Although the detection limit was supposed to be 6 Mb, the smallest fragment detected in this study was reported as 2.8 Mb, suggesting that detection sensitivity could be chromosome region dependent. Despite the fact that the sampling methods included polar bodies, blastomeres, and trophectoderm samples, the WGA efficiency was high (91.8% overall). Both CGH and aCGH were used for detection, and 77.7% of the samples were found to be chromosomally abnormal. Only 22.3% of samples were transferable, however, and a notable observation was that a significant proportion of the embryos were carrying abnormalities unrelated to the rearrangement. That is, 28.9% displayed *de novo* aneuploidy although being normal/balanced, and 27.3% were both unbalanced and aneuploid. The CPR per ET was 45.5% (26.4% per treatment cycle) and the delivery rate per ET was 27%. Although the pregnancy rate was not markedly increased in this study, no miscarriages were reported [81]. A later study [80] analyzed 34 couples in 50 cycles with rearrangements, including 9 RobT, 21 reciprocal translocations, 2 inversions, 1 insertional translocation, and 1 complex translocation. After blastocyst biopsy, 35.7% of embryos were found to be euploid or normal/balanced for the rearrangement, and 64.3% were abnormal. Of the 133 abnormal embryos, 36.1% carried an unbalanced rearrangement that was related to the parental abnormality. A combination of unbalanced parentally derived rearrangements and chromosome abnormalities not related to the rearrangement was seen in 20.3% of the embryos, and 34.6% of abnormal embryos were diagnosed with chromosome abnormality not related to parental translocation. The live birth rate (LBR) per ET was 31.7%.

In order to assess the origin of additional aneuploidies unrelated to the translocation, Ghevaria and colleagues, followed up embryos after they had been diagnosed as abnormal at cleavage stage by the aCGH technique [57]. According to their initial results, 55%–65% of cleavage-stage embryos displayed additional aneuploidies unrelated to the translocation. Abnormal blastocysts were followed up (day 5–7) and embryos diagnosed as aneuploid (by aCGH) were analyzed using FISH. Subsequent analysis of embryos with FISH demonstrated that meiotic aneuploidy affected 35% of embryos, 47% displayed a mitotic event, and 15% had both types. Of the 256 embryos that were diagnosed as untransferable, 63% carried additional aneuploidies.

Overall, therefore, aCGH was a successful era for PGT-SR, increasing clinical pregnancy rate from 40% (when using FISH) [6] to 70% [76]. Because of the "noisy" nature of the aCGH traces produced, inability to detect low level mosaicism and the cost of the test however, the use of aCGH was short lived and was superseded by SNP arrays (e.g., karyomapping) and NGS.

SNP Arrays and Karyomapping

A single-nucleotide polymorphism (SNP) is a DNA variant, occurring in ~1/1000 nucleotides. For PGT-SR diagnosis, a SNP microarray typically consists of ~300,000 features evenly distributed throughout the genome [82]. The assessment of parental DNA follows the deduction of four parental haplotypes for each chromosomal region and allows the detection of parental origin of chromosomal abnormalities. With SNP arrays, the polymorphic genotypes (AA, AB, BB) are analyzed for each sample and compared with the human haplotype map (HapMap) reference. The array features on an SNP array are more numerous and hence denser than those on an aCGH array. This provides a higher resolution, but their smaller size can cause poorer hybridization efficiencies, or no-calls. SNP arrays were validated by Treff and colleagues, first for whole chromosomal aneuploidy [83], then later for segmental imbalances [84]. SNP arrays generate both qualitative and quantitative data, and thus not only test for simultaneous detection of segmental imbalances and *de novo* aneuploidies of chromosomes not involved in the translocation, but can also distinguish balanced translocation carriers and normal embryos [82,85,86]. The only limitation is the availability of parental DNA, and at least one unbalanced embryo is needed to make the approach applicable to the majority of carrier couples [87]. In order to distinguish between carrier and normal embryo however, informative SNPs within 5 Mb of the breakpoints on each of the two chromosomes involved in the translocation are identified by analysis of parental DNA, then a comparison of the genotypes at these informative SNP positions are performed for each balanced/normal embryo against all possible unbalanced embryos [86]. Another advantage of SNP arrays is that they can also detect UPD.

Developed as a universal test for PGT, karyomapping for PGT-M and PGT-A is covered in other chapters in this book; its application for PGT-SR was immediately evident from the first studies [82]. Unique traces for normal, balanced carrier and unbalanced embryos were apparent from the outset, not only in karyomapping but also similar approaches such as haplarithmisis and the more recently described preimplantation genetic haplotyping, BasePhasing [88,89]. The specifics of the various approaches using SNP data for PGT-SR are described next.

Treff et al. analyzed 18 couples carrying either RecT or RobT. Trophectoderm biopsy preceded SNP array analysis with an IR of 45% and a CPR per ET of 75% [84]. This study provided the first opportunity to improve outcomes through comprehensive chromosome screening of euploid embryos from translocation carrier parents. It also highlighted the value of simultaneous aneuploidy screening. Out of 122 blastocysts, 62 (50.8%) were normal or balanced; among the remainder, 23 were aneuploid for at least one chromosome not associated with the translocation. van Uum et al. [90] analyzed 36 cleavage-stage embryos, dissociated after being initially diagnosed as unbalanced by FISH. SNP array results showed poor correlation with the initial FISH diagnosis: 64% were confirmed, 14% were found to be balanced (contrary to the initial diagnosis), and 22% were mosaic, probably due to the differences in technical and sampling methods used in this study [90]. Tan et al., in a retrospective study, compared the clinical effectiveness of SNP array analysis on day 5 embryos with FISH analysis at cleavage stage [91]. Using an SNP array achieved higher implantation rates (69% vs. 38% for RobT, 74% vs. 39% for RecT) (p < 0.001) and lower miscarriage rates than the FISH approach. Compared with FISH, SNP-based PGT-SR could identify >15% more chromosomal abnormalities unrelated to the translocation. Despite this, the percentage of transferable embryos was higher in SNP-based PGT-SR for both RobT and RecT (p > 0.001) probably due to more accurate diagnosis of SNP technique and the influence of biopsy stage where blastocysts are more likely to be chromosomally normal than cleavage-stage embryos [91]. Indeed, many studies have indicated that array-based PGT-SR of translocation carriers can lead to CPR of 45%–70% per ET [76,79,84,90]. In a retrospective study comparing aCGH and SNP-array platforms [92], both cleavage-stage and blastocyst-stage embryos from reciprocal translocation carriers were analyzed. Significant differences were observed between SNP and aCGH when analyzing the prevalence of embryos that were euploid and balanced/normal, but the clinical pregnancy rates were equivalent for SNP (60%) versus aCGH (65%). Overall, out of 498 embryos analyzed, 45% were euploid and balanced, 24% were balanced for the translocation chromosomes but aneuploid elsewhere, 23% contained only unbalanced translocation chromosomes, and 8% were both unbalanced and aneuploid. Overall SNP arrays detected 47% of embryos as euploid and balanced, whereas the figure was 39% of the embryos using aCGH. Combining both techniques, there was a significant difference in the aneuploidy rates between cleavage-stage embryos (38%) and blastocyst stage (22%) overall (p < 0.001). They demonstrated 22% increase in CPR compared to historical FISH testing (62% vs. 40%) [6]. Xiong and colleagues analyzed 169 couples (52 RobT, 117 RecT carriers): 23% of resultant embryos with RobT were unbalanced, whereas 52% of RecT were unbalanced. Nineteen percent of embryos from RobT and 12% from RecT were found to have *de novo* aneuploidies unrelated to the translocation [93]. Idowu and colleagues analyzed 74 couples, finding a statistical difference in the rate of unbalanced embryos between male and female translocation carriers (12% vs. 24%, $p < 0.05$) [94]. The rates of unbalanced embryos did not differ between day 3 and day 5 biopsy groups and between maternal age groups; yet, euploidy rates were lower for maternal age ≥ 35 group compared to <35, (19% vs. 29%, $p < 0.05$) and blastocyst embryos were more likely to be euploid than cleavage-stage embryos (42% vs. 22%, $p < 0.05$). In this study, the LBR reported per cycle with biopsy and per cycle with transfer were 38% and 52% respectively, which were higher than previously reported. Wang and colleagues analyzed 55 cycles for RobT and 181 cycles for RecT [95]. Using a regression model, they showed that three factors significantly affected the number of genetically transferable embryos: number of biopsied embryos ($p = 0.001$), basal FSH level ($p = 0.040$), and maternal age ($p = 0.027$). In their studies, they have found a normal/balanced rate of 42.2% in RobT and 26.9% in RecT, compared to Idowu and colleagues who showed 37% RobT and 19% RecT using the same array and approach [94,95]. In both studies, CPR per ET was similar (44.2% vs. 42.6%). Zhang and colleagues looked at 11 translocation families, analyzing 68 blastocysts, for which 42 were unbalanced or aneuploid and the remaining 26 were balanced or normal. In this study, 13 embryos were transferred and followed up by amniocentesis (which corroborated the initial diagnosis) [88]. More recently, Zhang and colleagues used BasePhasing in 2 balanced translocation families and 18 blastocysts in which 8 were unbalanced and the remaining 10 were balanced or normal [89]. Two embryo transfers ensued, corroborated by amniocentesis. Kubicek and colleagues used similar approaches to determine that segmental aneuploidies predominantly affect paternally derived chromosomes, while Beyer and colleagues, in a single case report, used karyomapping for PGT-SR, determining it to be feasible to distinguish normal/balanced outcomes from all unbalanced outcomes reliably [96,97]. A clinical pregnancy was achieved; in addition, addition, this technique allowed high-resolution analysis, with the smallest fragment detected in this case being 659 kb [97].

Taking all the studies together, the SNP-based approach has been an effective tool for PGT-SR with the advantage over other approaches of being able to detect balanced translocation carrier embryos. The question of whether balanced carriers *should* be screened and not transferred is another discussion and sometimes a requirement, especially when balanced translocation is associated with a genetic syndrome [85] (also discussed in elsewhere in this chapter).

Next-Generation Sequencing

Next-generation sequencing (NGS) is a very powerful approach for PGT-SR, involving parallel sequencing of whole or a targeted region of the genome, the use of a DNA barcoding system to identify individual samples (thereby allowing multiple samples to be run in one reaction), and complex bioinformatic analysis to "bin" each sequence by chromosome location, thereby permitting quantitative analysis [98]. In recent years, the cost of equipment and reagents has fallen rapidly and thereby increased the usage and the popularity of this approach. The advantage of this technique is that it is easy, accessible, low cost, and high throughput. It has several technical advantages over other means of cytogenetic detection such as simultaneous testing for aneuploidy, segmental imbalances, and mitochondrial DNA analysis; it also has a greater dynamic range for the detection of mosaicism [99,100].

Like CGH, aCGH, and SNP arrays, NGS requires a prior WGA step (see Chapter 3 for detail). There are two main NGS platforms currently being used for PGT-SR—semiconductor sequencing, which is based on the detection of hydrogen ions that are released during the polymerization of DNA (Ion Torrent, Thermo-Fisher Scientific), and Illumina sequencing, which is based on sequencing by synthesis with fluorescently labeled reversible terminators (VeriSeq, Illumina). The sensitivity and specificity of those methods are different and depends on coverage and the sequencing depth.

The most important consideration is the resolution of each platform to detect small segmental imbalances (reviewed [101]), although this is influenced by the location of the chromosomal region. The resolution of aCGH has been reported as between 2.5 and 2.8 Mb [76,81], SNP arrays as 2.4 Mb [85] and, originally, the ion torrent sequencing method as 5–6 Mb [102]. Cuman and colleagues compared the resolution of aCGH versus VeriSeq NGS for the detection of segmental imbalances [103]. In 200 WGA products of embryos from rearrangement carriers, 100% concordance was established. NGS was able to detect 97%

of the unbalanced segments previously identified using aCGH; however, 20% of segmental imbalances smaller than 20 Mb could not be detected by NGS. Therefore, the authors concluded that aCGH remained the gold standard and, for both reciprocal translocation and inversion carriers, a minimum of three out of four segments must be >10 Mb to ensure accurate diagnosis with NGS. Yin and colleagues compared the HighSeq2000 platform (Illumina) with the Affymetrix SNP array on 38 biopsies, demonstrating a greater accuracy in some genomic regions using NGS [104]. Moreover, Tan and colleagues provided the first evaluation of clinical outcome of NGS based PGT-A and PGT-SR, also comparing the efficiencies of SNP-array and NGS and finding that NGS was able to detect some segmental imbalances not detected by SNP array [105].

Gui and colleagues compared the diagnostic efficiencies of cleavage-stage FISH and the blastocyst stage of the corresponding embryos from rearrangement carriers by NGS (HiSeq 2500 platform, Illumina) [106]. The smallest fragment detected by NGS was 5.1 Mb. According to their results, only 62% of rearrangement-associated chromosomes showed consistency between cleavage-stage FISH and blastocyst-stage NGS. More strikingly, the majority of inconsistencies (87.5%) were found in embryos that were diagnosed as "unbalanced" by cleavage-stage FISH but "balanced" by blastocyst-stage NGS. The authors suggested genetic mosaicism and/or FISH artefacts as possible reasons for these inconsistencies. This study demonstrated that old methods of both genetic testing (FISH) and sampling (blastomere biopsy) were inaccurate, and blastocyst-stage biopsy followed by NGS-based analysis should be recommended for PGT-SR going forward [106]. Chow and colleagues examined concordance between aCGH (24Sure+, Illumina) and NGS (VeriSeq-PGS MiSeq, Illumina) in 342 embryos from 41 rearrangement carriers (38 RecT and 3 inversions). A total of 87 blastomere and 55 trophectoderm biopsied showed 100% concordant results although some segments <10 Mb were detected by aCGH but not by NGS. Furthermore, in their study, an imbalance with a 534-kb fragment was detected by aCGH [107].

Zhang and colleagues provided some of the first clinical experience with a novel high-resolution NGS for PGT-SR, which they named copy number variation sequencing (CNV-Seq) using the HighSeq 2500 platform [108]. Two key modifications from the existing platforms were that: they used threefold higher mapped sequencing reads that were binned at smaller intervals (20 kb). Embryos (24 cleavage stage and 74 blastocyst stage) from 21 couples (4 RobT and 17 RecT) revealed that 30.6% were balanced for all chromosomes, 20.4% were balanced for the rearranged but aneuploid for another chromosome, 33.7% were unbalanced, 15.3% were both unbalanced and aneuploid. The main advantage of this approach is its high resolution, making it possible to detect imbalanced hitherto not reported for any other platform (as low as 0.8 Mb) as well as a better detection of mosaicism (down to 20%). Most recently, Wang and colleagues analyzed 378 blastocyst-stage embryos from 89 patients with RecT, finding 32.3% normal or balanced. The largest clinical study to date, it reported clinical pregnancy rates of 70.5% and live birth rates of 65.9% per blastocyst transfer using the NGS technique [109].

When comparing different NGS platforms for PGT-SR (and for the detection of segmental imbalance generally), there is clearly antagonism between the cost of the test and the resolution, with lower coverage platforms that are easily applicable, high throughput, and cost effective, and higher resolution methods offering a better resolution both for size of the fragment (e.g., for cryptic translocations) and the level of mosaicism, but they are at a price. Nonetheless, the ability of NGS to produce large amounts of data, the increasing availability and cost-effectiveness of the approach, plus its now-increased sensitivity compared to older methodologies, make NGS the method of choice for PGT-SR. Nevertheless, the best platform to use depends on the size of the segments, chromosomal region, and the sampling method (blastomere, trophectoderm, or spent culture media), since the amount of genetic material also limits the resolution of each technique significantly. For a comparison of technical methods and a summary of clinical outcomes, see Tables 4.2 and 4.3.

Discussion

PGT-SR is a multidisciplinary task with the ultimate goal of helping those carrier couples to have a chromosomally normal or at least chromosomally "balanced" (e.g., carrier) child. In this context, there are both clinical and genetic factors affecting the outcome of the treatment cycles herein discussed.

TABLE 4.2

Comparison of Techniques Used in PGT-SR

Detection Parameters/ Techniques	FISH	aCGH	SNP Array/ Karyomapping	NGS
Resolution of detection of inherited segmental abnormalities[a]/the smallest fragment detected for imbalances in the literature	50–100 Kb	~5 Mb/ 0.6–2.5 Mb [76,79,107]	~5–10 Mb/0.7–2.36 Mb [85,91,97]	~5–10 Mb/~0,8–2 Mb [102,103,108]
Simultaneous CCS (24-chromosome testing)	–	+	+	+
Detection of *de novo* segmental abnormalities	–	+	+	+
Need for WGA (whole-genome amplification)	–	+	+	+
Need for preclinical workup	+	–	+	–
Need for analysis of parental/ grandparental DNA	+	–	+	–
Ability to distinguish normal from balanced	–	–	+	–[b]

[a] According to the product information provided by the manufacturer, the reliable resolution of detection of those techniques may differ according to the genomic region and the type of biopsy material.

[b] Only with special mate-pair NGS protocol [110].

Factors Affecting Meiotic Segregational Patterns and the Availability of Normal/Balanced and Euploid Embryos

Prediction of the segregation patterns of chromosomes for PGT-SR is invaluable in the context of genetic counseling and future planning for patients in order to foresee the risks involved in the treatment. It is well known that the probability of alternate segregation in RobT is much higher than in RecT (theoretically 1/4 vs. 1/8; see Introduction part); thus the translocation types are the major determining factor in the proportion of normal/balanced embryos. Besides the translocation types, meiotic segregation modes were analyzed in several studies to investigate whether the sex of the carrier, presence of terminal breakpoints, and the chromosomal types involved in translocation affect meiotic segregations and the proportion of normal/balanced embryos [60,61,111–115].

Involvement of acrocentric chromosomes in RecT seems to have a negative impact on the rate of 2:2 segregations. Using FISH on blastomeres, several studies reported that the incidence of alternative segregation was significantly lower in RecT carriers associated with acrocentric chromosomes (13, 14, 15, 21, 22) when compared to those without (for instance (14.6% acrocentric vs. 26.0% others) in one study [60], and (39.2% acrocentric vs. 60.2% others) in another study [112]; p = 0.001 in both cases). The authors stated that the relatively unstable nature of acrocentric chromosomes compared with (sub)metacentric chromosomes might be responsible for a possible disruption of quadrivalent structure increasing the proportion of abnormal meiotic segregational products. Similarly, using NGS method on blastocysts revealed that, the proportion of alternate segregation involving acrocentric chromosomes was lower than that of blastocysts from RecT carriers without acrocentric chromosomes. Translocations with acrocentric chromosomes exhibited a significantly higher incidence of 3:1 segregation [109]. Furthermore, there is some evidence that the effects of acrocentric chromosomes on segregations might be sex-specific. More recently, with aCGH technology (see previous sections and Chapter 3), meiotic segregation patterns of 2101 blastocysts from 243 female carriers, including 76 cases with translocations involving acrocentric chromosomes, and 230 male carriers, including 88 cases with translocations involving acrocentric chromosomes, were analyzed according to chromosome type, carrier sex, and age. In cases with translocations involving the acrocentric chromosomes subgroup, the proportion of alternate segregation (53.9% vs. 33.4%, p < 0.0001) was significantly higher in male carriers than in female carriers, with the proportion of 3:1 segregation (6.8% vs. 16.3%, p < 0.0001) being significantly lower [115].

TABLE 4.3

Summary of Clinical Outcomes in PGT-SR

Study	No of Cycles/ Embryos Analyzed	Rearrangement Type (No of Patients/Cycles Where Available)	Female Age (Mean)	Biopsy Material	Technique	Normal/ Balanced and Euploid (Transferable) (%)	CPR per ET (%)	IR per ET (%)	LBR per ET (%)
Kuliev et al. [59]	475/3825	361 RecT 90 RobT 24 Others	–	Polar body (19.3%) Blastomere (80.7%)	FISH	23.6% in RecT 42.3% in RobT	38	–	26.9
Ko et al. [61]	133/1508	RecT	32.1 ± 3.6	Blastomere	FISH	18.7	28.4	–	20.7
Keymolen et al. [64]	312/1553	RecT	32.8 ± 4.3	Blastomere	FISH	20.8	36.7[a]	–	26.7
Harper et al. [6]	4253/24773	1213 RobT 2413 RecT 627 Others	–	Blastomere (in the majority of the cases)	FISH	26	26	–	–
Alwarati et al. [81]	20/121	5 RobT, 9 RecT, 2 Inv	36.3	PBs, blastomeres, trophectoderm	CGH/ aCGH	22.3	45.5	–	27
Fiorentino et al. [76]	28/187	8 RobT	38.0 ± 2.1	Blastomere	aCGH	27.5	83.3	66.7	–
		16 Rec	37.1 ± 3.7	Blastomere	aCGH	11.8	63.6	61.5	–
Tan et al. [91]	52/218	52 RobT	31.7 ± 5.02	Trophectoderm	SNP	58	69	52	–
	149/1204	149 RobT	30.8 ± 3.97	Blastomere	FISH	36	38	28	–
	117/499	117 RecT	30.8 ± 4.74	Trophectoderm	SNP	36	74	59	–
	257/2258	257 RecT	29.9 ± 3.67	Blastomere	FISH	20	39	32	–
Tan et al. [105]	129/454	18 RobT 59 RecT 7 Inv 45 AMA/RM	33.6	Trophectoderm	NGS	43.6	61.3	52.6	–
	266/1058	58 RobT 144 RecT 11 Inv 53 AMA/RM	31.4	Trophectoderm	SNP-array	44.2	56.7	47.6	
Tobler et al. [92]	58/396	47 RecT	34.3 ± 4.2	Blastomere (68%) Trophectoderm (32%)	SNP-array	47	60	–	–
	17/102	16 RecT	32 ± 3.3	Blastomere (57%) Trophectoderm (43%)	aCGH	39	65	–	–
Christodoulou et al. [80]	50/207	21 RecT, 9 RobT, 2 inv, 1 insT, 1 complex T	32.5 (26–40)	Trophectoderm	aCGH	35.7	43.9	30.2	31.7
Idowu et al. [94]	32/201	32 RobT	33.9	Blastomere (81.1%) Trophectoderm (18.9%)	SNP-array	37	56	–	52
	42/338	42 RecT	34.0			19	59	–	52
Zhang et al. [108]	21 /98	4 RobT 17 RecT	32.5 (25–39)	Blastomere, Trophectoderm	NGS, (CNV-Seq)	30.6	–	80.0	70.0
Wang et al. [109]	102/378	89 RecT	28.8 ± 3.5	Trophectoderm	NGS	32.3	70.5	–	65.9

Notes: Only reports that provide clinical data are included.

Clinical outcomes were given separately for each rearrangement group where available.

[a] Based on positive hCG and not fetal heartbeat.

The sex of the carrier seems to have an impact on the segregational outcomes for both RobT and RecT, in the advantage of male carriers. Specifically, 2:2 segregations were significantly higher in males than in female carriers (60.8% vs. 52.7%, p < 0.05) and accordingly, the incidence of 3:1 and 4:0 segregations were significantly higher in female (p < 0.05) than in male carriers [61]. The proportion of normal/balanced embryos in male RecT carriers were higher than in female RecT carriers (35.5% vs. 23.8%) and the proportion of 3:1 segregation was the predominant mode in female carriers (31%), yet it did not reach statistical significance, possibly due to low sample size (14 couples) [111]. Another study also revealed that the incidence of 2:2 segregation was significantly higher in male than in female carriers (58.2% vs. 45.0%, p = 0.019) [112]. Chang et al. analyzed outcomes of 66 cycles of 34 RobT carrier couples in which 514 blastomeres were tested and they found a higher proportion of normal or balanced embryos in couples with male carriers (32.1%) than those with female carriers (27.7%); nevertheless, sex did not have any impact on the clinical outcomes [113]. More recently with aCGH, 154 couples with RobT (77 male and 77 female carriers; 172 cycles) were tested and 604 blastocysts were analyzed [114]. The frequencies of alternate, adjacent, and 3:0 segregation patterns were 68.0%, 30.6%, and 1.3%, respectively. The proportion of alternate segregation was significantly higher (82.9% vs. 55.2%, p < 0.001) in male carriers than in female carriers. This sex-linked selective process against unbalanced segregational products might be due to relatively less strict checkpoint in female gametogenesis [116], where the arrest of the division results in the elimination of unbalanced segregation in spermatogenesis [114].

The position of the breakpoint is another parameter that could affect the segregational products. According to the meiotic segregation patterns of 278 embryos obtained from 41 PGT-SR cycles for RecT carriers, the incidence of normal/balanced embryos in RecT with terminal breakpoints was significantly lower than those without (6.5% vs. 14.4%, p = 0.005) [112]. In contrast, in another recently published study, the rate of alternate segregation in RecT with terminal breakpoints was not different from that in RecT without terminal breakpoints; however, the frequency of adjacent-2 segregation was significantly different between two groups (6.7% vs. 15.5%, p = 0.013) [109].

Biopsy stage and maternal age do not seem to have a strong effect on the segregational patterns; however, they affect the proportion of transferable embryos. Euploidy rates were significantly lower in couples with advanced compared to young maternal age, respectively [114,117]. Beyer and colleagues demonstrated an increase in the proportion of genetically normal/balanced embryos on day 5/6 of development, which they suggested was due to a strong selection process between day 3 and day 5/6 in favor of normal/balanced embryos [21]. In RecT carriers, the rate of alternate segregation in day 3 embryos (22.3%) was lower compared to day 5/6 (53.1%, p < 0.0001). Similarly, in the RobT group, the rate of alternate segregation was significantly lower on day 3 compared to day 5/6 embryos (38.7% vs. 74.1, p < 0.0001). In another study, performed by comprehensive chromosome screening techniques, Xie et al. demonstrated that the rate of euploid and balanced/normal embryos was significantly lower in cleavage stage compared to blastocyst stage in both RecT and RobT carrier embryos [117]. However, those segregational differences reported here might be caused by the differences in the overall aneuploidy rates between blastocyst stage and cleavage stage where post meiotic abnormalities are seen more often, dominating over the abnormalities related to translocation itself.

The Interchromosomal Effect

Put simply, an interchromosomal effect (ICE) is where the presence of one chromosome abnormality (e.g., perpetuated by a translocation) makes the presence of further chromosome abnormalities (e.g., *de novo* aneuploidy) more likely. Studies of PGT-SR have allowed investigation of the ICE in early human development. The ICE was first postulated by Lejeune, and then Lindenbaum, who observed that there was a higher risk of having children with Down syndrome among carriers of rearrangements [118,119]. Although it remains a subject of controversy, ICE can be explained by the possible impact of rearranged chromosomes on the segregations, pairing, and disjunction of other chromosomes during meiosis resulting in the elevated risk of production of aneuploid gametes via heterosynapsis between translocated chromosomes and sex vesicle [120] or disruption in chromosomal positions and territorials [121]. This phenomenon of ICE has been studied extensively in sperm samples as well as in embryos of carrier couples; however, results are highly variable and controversial. Sperm karyotyping studies have not shown any support for ICE in translocations and inversions [31]. However, an evidence of ICE in rearrangement carriers with poor sperm morphology has been proposed [122]. Segregation patterns of 10 chromosomes (1, 4, 9, 13, 15, 16, 20, 21, X, Y) by FISH from 9 carriers and compared with 3 normal men revealed no evidence of an ICE in fertile carriers, whereas significant variations were observed in all chromosomes tested in the group of infertile translocation carriers, suggesting a correlation between poor quality spermatozoa and increased aneuploidy rate in this group [122]. In RecT heterozygotes, abnormal semen profiles were much more common among the cases demonstrating an interchromosomal effect (67%) compared with those that did not (11%) (reviewed [25]). Therefore, it is possible that ICE might be patient specific and related to infertility factors rather than the rearrangement itself [25]. Furthermore, ICE might also be chromosome specific; six male carriers were analyzed for chromosomes 1, 15, 16, 17, 18, X, and Y, and increased disomy rates were found only in three of the six chromosomes analyzed for aneuploidy and not in others [146].

A recent study [123] drew attention to the combined presence of both aneuploidy and segregation abnormalities in the same sperm. This study is important in that it is the first to analyze both segregation analysis and aneuploidy testing (13, 18, 21, X, Y) on the same spermatozoa [123]. Aneuploid sperm displayed significant decreases in the 2:2 alternate segregation (21.8%) versus non-selected spermatozoa (43.8%), which showed for RecT carriers that the vast majority of the spermatozoa with *de novo* numerical abnormalities also display an unbalanced segregation content of the rearranged chromosomes, which could imply a wide general failure in meiosis I [123].

There are also conflicting results in the studies on preimplantation embryos. Gianaroli and colleagues suggested that an ICE might be the responsible mechanism that increases the proportion of abnormal embryos in RobT but not in RecT carriers [62], whereas other studies have not found any evidence of ICE in embryos [55,124,125,127,128].

Interestingly, a study suggested that RobT could trigger an ICE by inducing genetic instability in early mitotic divisions [129] in embryos from female carriers [130]. According to the comprehensive chromosomal analysis of 283 samples, including oocytes and early embryos from 44 patients by aCGH, although small, an increased risk of aneuploidy compared to clinically matched non-translocation carrier couples was found (0.4% per chromosome, $p < 0.0001$). However, this effect was observed only at cleavage stage, suggesting a mitotic rather than a meiotic origin [130]. In addition, the same effect was not observed in the embryos of RecT and inversion carriers. In a recent study with the comparison of control group, no ICE was observed in either cleavage- or blastocyst-stage embryos from RecT nor RobT carriers [117]. Also, in line with RecT and RobT, an ICE was not observed in embryos from heterozygote inversion carriers such that the incidence of aneuploidy was not significantly higher for the inversion patients compared to the controls (inversion = 48.8% vs. control = 47.2% ns) [128].

For now, there is no consensus on whether or not rearrangements affect the segregation of other chromosomes, and the presence of an ICE in IVF embryos is still under debate.

Embryonic Developmental Characteristics and Ovarian Response in Carriers

There is a strong correlation between gross chromosomal errors and delayed/arrested embryonic development [131,132]. The existence of such a correlation raised the question of whether it might be used as an indicator to help to distinguish unbalanced embryos from balanced ones in early preimplantation development. In a retrospective study where the ability of an embryo to reach to the blastocyst stage was the main observation, no evident selection against chromosomally unbalanced embryos was found, which showed the segmental imbalances due to rearrangements do not affect the embryo's ability to reach blastocyst stage [133]. Another study found no difference between the morphological characteristics of normal/balanced and unbalanced embryos [113]. In contrast to previous results, Treff and colleagues observed developmental differences between unbalanced embryos normal/balanced ones, such that; arrested embryos were significantly more likely to possess unbalanced chromosomes when compared with developmentally competent blastocysts ($p < 0.05$); suggesting that preimplantation embryo development might be impacted negatively by the presence of unbalanced derivative chromosomes [84]. Findikli and colleagues compared the developmental characteristics of embryos of translocation carriers with those of standard IVF patients. The rate of blastocyst formation was not different between unbalanced and balanced/normal embryos in the carrier group, which is in line with a few other studies [113,133]; however, overall significant differences were observed in translocation carrier's embryos compared to non-translocation cases, in terms of fertilization rates, embryo development, and blastocyst formation (16.1% for RecT, 26.1% for RobT, 41.9% for standard ICSI cycles, respectively) [134]. Despite this, it was not possible to draw firm conclusions on this topic due to the low sample size, where only nine reciprocal and six RobT carriers were included in this study.

After the development of time-lapse technology (see Chapter 10 in this book), precise cell cycle parameter timing and detailed information on the morphokinetic behavior of embryos is now available. There is some evidence that euploid and aneuploid embryos follow different morphokinetic behaviors [135], and some morphokinetic parameters were found to be correlated with implantation [136]. However, not only numerical abnormalities but also segmental imbalances seem to influence morphokinetic parameters. Time-lapse imaging revealed that embryos carrying unbalanced translocations exhibit a delay in time of cleavage to the four-cell stage (defined as t4,38.22 h vs. 39.49 h) and in time of the start of blastulation (tSB; 100.14 h vs. 103.71 h), and embryos with unbalanced forms of translocations mainly of maternal origin have been shown to be delayed in certain morphokinetic parameters (tPNf,t2,t3,t4,t6,t7,t8,cc2,s2, and tSB) compared to balanced embryos ($p < 0.05$) [138]. However, since the diagnosis is based on the FISH technique with cleavage-stage biopsy, additional aneuploidy testing was not available, so whether they are pure unbalanced embryos or also carrying additional aneuploidy is unknown. Another study compared morphokinetic parameters of 177 balanced embryos with 250 unbalanced embryos using time-lapse technology [139]. Although significant differences exist between balanced and unbalanced embryos in translocation carriers in some of the parameters (t5,t9,cc2,s2, and t5-t2) ($p < 0.05$), none of the parameters were able to predict the chromosomal status of the embryo [139]. Although differences in some parameters do exist, for now, time-lapse technology should not be used as a diagnostic tool for chromosomal status in translocation carriers.

There are contradictory results on the possible association between female chromosome translocations and poor response to ovarian stimulation. The levels of estradiol (E2) on the day of human chorionic gonadotropin (hCG) administration in 61 cycles in 46 women with balanced translocations were compared with 42 cycles in 32 women whose male partner had a balanced translocation [140]. A significantly higher proportion of female carriers (23%) responded very poorly to ovarian stimulation compared to women whose partner carries the translocation (7%), suggesting that the ovarian response to gonadotropin stimulation might be negatively affected in female carriers. The study reveals that although not all patients carrying translocation are expected to have a poor response, some of them might be at increased risk based on individual biological differences [140]. The authors suggest an aggressive stimulation protocol where there is no ovarian hyperstimulation syndrome risk for these low responders.

In contrast, Dechanet and colleagues analyzed the clinical data of 79 cycles from 33 female translocation carriers and compared them with 116 cycles from 55 male carriers. No difference was observed for the following controlled ovarian stimulation (COS) parameters: total dose of recombinant FSH and the number of retrieved oocytes and embryos on day 3. Pregnancy rates were also similar ($p = 0.28$). This study showed that the ovarian response to COS was not impaired by the balanced translocation status. Therefore, authors suggest that female carriers of balanced chromosome rearrangements could be considered as normal responders [141].

Deselection of Carrier Embryos

Although it is assumed that "balanced rearrangements" incur no gain or loss of the genetic material, this may not always be the case. With the aid of recent technological improvements such as combination of paired-end whole-genome sequencing and Sanger sequencing, it is possible to characterize translocation and inversion breakpoints at single base-pair resolution [142,143]. Those studies suggest that although the translocation may seem balanced, often there are some additional or missing nucleotides as a result of an imprecise non-homologous end joining process, which in some cases may result in the manifestation of a disease phenotype [143] in so-called balanced carriers. This is often a risk for *de novo* translocation carriers where the consequences of this "balanced" translocation is not known. Besides the transmission of those rearrangements, knowing that they might cause the same reproductive problems makes the deselection of carrier embryos more preferable. The rationale is to ensure their child will not be faced with the same reproductive problems, such as infertility and recurrent miscarriages. Initially, FISH with breakpoint spanning probes were used to differentiate between normal and carrier embryos [53]. Another approach was nuclear conversion technique [59]; however, both techniques were time consuming, and the design of specific probes for each case is not feasible.

Sometimes the deselection of carrier embryos is necessary, especially when there is a genetic risk associated with the translocation [85]. In 2011, the first clinical case of microarray-based PGT-SR being used to distinguish between carrier and normal chromosomes was reported for that reason. With the use of SNP-array platform, Treff and colleagues have successfully distinguished carrier embryos obtained from a 28-year-old patient with Alagille syndrome which was caused by an apparently balanced translocation of 46,XX,t(2;20)(q21;p12.2). This translocation caused a microdeletion on the short arm of chromosome 20, disrupting Jagged1 gene [85,144]. Then the same group reported their retrospective analysis of 126 embryos evaluated as normal/carrier in the regular PGT-SR study. After carrier diagnosis, 62 were predicted to be normal (49%), and 64 (51%) were predicted as balanced [86]. In order to distinguish normal from balanced, the only prerequisite is that it is necessary to have parental DNA, and the presence of unbalanced embryos. This works in three phases: (i) informative SNPs within 5 Mb of the breakpoints on each of the two chromosomes are identified on parental DNA; (ii) comprehensive chromosome screening on embryo biopsies is performed (unbalanced embryos serve as linkage analysis); and (iii) the normal/balanced embryos are evaluated according to the information gathered from unbalanced embryo genotypes. This method relies on the availability of the presence of unbalanced embryos. In these studies, the implantation potentials of carrier versus normal embryos were not different ($p = 0.33$).

Later, using an NGS platform, Hu and colleagues developed a technique called micro-SeqPGD, where the derivative chromosomes were micro-dissected from G-banded metaphase spreads of the patients' peripheral bloods [145]. The dissected fragments were amplified by degenerate oligonucleotide-primed PCR (DOP-PCR). Breakpoint mapping was based on parallel sequencing with paired-end protocol and a bespoke bioinformatic analysis, and informative SNPs were identified flanking the breakpoints. Precise characterization of breakpoints was confirmed by Sanger sequencing. In the PGT-SR study, the embryos that were diagnosed as normal/balanced by the initial NGS analysis were analyzed further with junction-specific primers and the SNP information obtained from preclinical workup. Out of 44 blastocysts from 8 couples, 15 were either normal/balanced and euploid [145]. Surprisingly, linkage analysis showed 13 of them were balanced, and only 2 were normal. The small sample size could be attributed for this bias in the proportion of normal versus carrier embryos.

Wang and colleagues developed a novel strategy using a combination of mate-pair sequencing and PCR breakpoint analysis of balanced translocation derivatives for distinguishing between carrier and normal embryos [110]. The breakpoints were successfully identified in only 9 patients out of 11 (82%). In two patients, they were not able to identify the breakpoints due to the presence of highly repetitive sequences in the proximal regions of the breakpoints. This study resulted in the birth of healthy girl with normal karyotype. There are some limitations of this technique. In cases where the breakpoints map to highly repetitive sequences or AT-rich sequence islands, this approach is not feasible. Moreover, the preclinical workup and the design of the experiments may take 1 month to complete, which is costly and labor-intensive.

The aforementioned methods require preclinical workup and thus are time consuming. As mentioned previously, techniques such as karyomapping, haplarithmisis, and chromosomal phasing on base level (BasePhasing) [82,88,89] distinguish normal from balanced carriers based on genome-wide genetic haplotyping analysis using an SNP microarray. Zhang and colleagues examined 11 families and 68 blastocysts of which 12 were balanced for the translocation and 14 were normal using the preimplantation genetic haplotyping technique [88]. There are several advantages of this method over preexisting ones, such that the presence of an unbalanced embryo could be used as a reference in this technique with no requirement to study family members. The other advantages of this technique include the fact that it is a universal method for any kind of rearrangement—not only RecT but also RobT—and inversions are able to be analyzed by this method along with the genetic screening of all 23 pairs of chromosomes, the total process takes only a few days, and recombination less than 1 Mb are also detectable by this method [88] which makes this technique more reliable in the diagnosis of carrier status. Recently, the same group [89] developed an improved protocol named "chromosomal phasing on base level" (BasePhasing), which uses a more dense SNP-array (Illumina Infinium Asian Screening Array-24 v1.0,ASA with ~700 K SNPs) and a specially phasing pipeline. This method is again based on a genome-wide haplotyping algorithm [82]. After validation studies using cell lines, they tested 18 blastocysts from two translocation carrier families in which 8 were balanced and the other 10 blastocysts were normal for the translocation. The authors claim that BasePhasing is one of the most suitable methods to distinguish normal embryos from balanced carriers in PGT-SR at present, but it still needs for further validation with a larger sample size and in different ethnicities.

Conclusions

PGT-SR is perhaps the less well known of all forms of PGT but nonetheless provides effective treatment for a large number of carrier couples to avoid repeated spontaneous abortions and the fear of having an affected child. The fact that the imbalance caused by abnormal segregation can lead to implantation failure, miscarriages, or affected offspring and moreover, that for some translocations very few or none of the conceptuses with imbalance can survive to term, means that it is likely to continue into the future. PGT-SR is necessary and effective, and has benefited from the technical advances of PGT-A.

The biggest limiting factor is the availability of normal/balanced embryo(s) which is highly affected by the type of translocation (RecT vs. RobT), the chromosomes involved (acrocentric vs. non-acrocentric), and the sex of the carrier; however, maternal age does not have any impact on segregational patterns but decreases the chances of an embryo transfer in any given PGT-SR cycle due to the higher incidence of *de novo* aneuploidies.

Various techniques are available in the diagnosis of imbalances such as FISH, SNP-based techniques, aCGH, and NGS. As with all PGT variants, there is a variety of embryo sampling methods, the most common still being invasive (trophectoderm biopsy), although noninvasive and less invasive sampling methods recently introduced into clinical practice seem promising. PGT-SR has evolved through the years from when the FISH technique was used in cleavage-stage embryos. Better clinical results have been achieved after the implementation of more automated comprehensive diagnostic chromosomal screening methods and the wider use of blastocyst-stage biopsy. The reduction of wastage of transferable embryos via use of more reliable diagnostic techniques, the use of less damaging biopsy methods, and simultaneous aneuploidy screening have increased the effectiveness of the technique and improved clinical outcomes. Although heterogenous, the reports on the genetic and clinical outcomes of rearrangement carriers provide an invaluable data set which could help clinicians and genetic counselors to give patients better counseling and information on their individual reproductive risks associated with their rearrangements.

REFERENCES

1. Weckselblatt B, Hermetz KE, Rudd MK. Unbalanced translocations arise from diverse mutational mechanisms including chromothripsis. *Genome Res.* Jul 2015;25(7):937–47.
2. De Braekeleer M, Dao TN. Cytogenetic studies in couples experiencing repeated pregnancy losses. *Hum Reprod.* Jul 1990;5(5):519–28.
3. De Braekeleer M, Dao TN. Cytogenetic studies in male infertility: A review. *Hum Reprod.* Feb 1991;6(2):245–50.
4. Shah K et al. The genetic basis of infertility. *Reproduction.* 2003;126:13–25.
5. Scriven PN et al. Benefits and drawbacks of preimplantation genetic diagnosis (PGD) for reciprocal translocations: Lessons from a prospective cohort study. *Eur J Hum Genet.* Oct 2013;21(10):1035–41.
6. Harper JC et al. The ESHRE PGD Consortium: 10 years of data collection. *Hum Reprod Update.* May–Jun 2012;18(3):234–47.
7. Griffin DK, Ogur C. Chromosomal analysis in IVF: Just how useful is it? *Reproduction.* Jul 2018;156(1):F29–50. Review.
8. Lieber MR. The mechanism of double-strand DNA break repair by the nonhomologous DNA end-joining pathway. *Annu Rev Biochem.* 2010;79:181–211.

9. Hurles ME, Lupski JR. Recombination hotspots in nonallelic homologous recombination. In: Lupski JR, Stankiewicz P (eds). *Genomic Disorders.* Humana Press. 2006; 341–55.

10. Ou ZZ et al. Partial 5p deletion and partial 5q duplication in a patient with multiple congenital anomalies: A two-step mechanism in chromosomal rearrangement mediated by non-allelic homologous recombination. *Cytogenet Genome Res.* 5 Oct, 2018;156:65–70.

11. Weterings E, van Gent DC. The mechanism of non-homologous end-joining: A synopsis of synapsis. *DNA Repair (Amst).* 2004;3:1425–35.

12. Lee JA, Carvalho CM, Lupski JR. A DNA replication mechanism for generating nonrecurrent rearrangements associated with genomic disorders. *Cell.* 28 Dec, 2007;131(7):1235–47.

13. Pellestor F. Chromothripsis: How does such a catastrophic event impact human reproduction? *Hum Reprod.* Mar 2014;29(3):388–93.

14. Inagaki H et al. Palindrome-mediated translocations in humans: A new mechanistic model for gross chromosomal rearrangements. *Front Genet.* 12 Jul, 2016;7:125.

15. Tucker JD. Low-dose ionizing radiation and chromosome translocations: A review of the major considerations for human biological dosimetry. *Mutat Res.* Sep–Oct 2008;659(3):211–20.

16. Hook EB et al. Inherited structural cytogenetic abnormalities detected incidentally in fetuses diagnosed prenatally: Frequency, parental-age associations, sex-ratio trends, and comparisons with rates of mutants. *Am J Hum Genet.* Mar 1984;36(2):422–43.

17. Beyazyurek C et al. Preimplantation genetic diagnosis (PGD) for extremes--successful birth after PGD for a consanguineous couple carrying an identical balanced reciprocal translocation. *Fertil Steril.* 1 May, 2010;93(7):2413.e1–5.

18. Ohye T et al. Paternal origin of the de novo constitutional t(11;22)(q23;q11). *Eur J Hum Genet.* Jul 2010;18(7):783–7.

19. Jacobs PA et al. Estimates of the frequency of chromosome abnormalities detectable in unselected newborns using moderate levels of banding. *J Med Genet.* Feb 1992;29(2):103–8.

20. Scriven PN, Handyside AH, Ogilvie CM. Chromosome translocations: Segregation modes and strategies for preimplantation genetic diagnosis. *Prenat Diagn.* Dec 1998;18(13):1437–49.

21. Beyer CE, Willats E. Natural selection between day 3 and day 5/6 PGD embryos in couples with reciprocal or Robertsonian translocations. *J Assist Reprod Genet.* Nov 2017;34(11):1483–92.

22. Martin RH. A detailed method for obtaining preparations of human sperm chromosomes. *Cytogenet Cell Genet.* 1983;35(4):252–6.

23. Lamotte A et al. Is sperm FISH analysis still useful for Robertsonian translocations? Meiotic analysis for 23 patients and review of the literature. *Basic Clin Androl.* 7 May, 2018;28:5.

24. Patassini C et al. Molecular karyotyping of human single sperm by array- comparative genomic hybridization. *PLOS ONE.* 2013;8(4):e60922.

25. Martin RH. Cytogenetic determinants of male fertility. *Hum Reprod Update.* Jul–Aug 2008;14(4):379–90.

26. Goldman AS, Hultén MA. Analysis of chiasma frequency and first meiotic segregation in a human male reciprocal translocation heterozygote, t(1;11)(p36.3;q13.1), using fluorescence in situ hybridisation. *Cytogenet Cell Genet.* 1993;63(1):16–23.

27. Escudero T et al. Predictive value of sperm fluorescence in situ hybridization analysis on the outcome of preimplantation genetic diagnosis for translocations. *Fertil Steril.* Jun 2003;79 Suppl 3:1528–34.

28. Luciani JM et al. Pachytene analysis of a man with a 13q;14q translocation and infertility. Behavior of the trivalent and nonrandom association with the sex vesicle. *Cytogenet Cell Genet.* 1984;38(1):14–22.

29. Pettenati MJ et al. Paracentric inversions in humans: A review of 446 paracentric inversions with presentation of 120 new cases. *Am J Med Genet.* 16 Jan, 1995;55(2):171–87.

30. Jaarola M, Martin RH, Ashley T. Direct evidence for suppression of recombination within two pericentric inversions in humans: A new sperm-FISH technique. *Am J Hum Genet.* 1998;63(1):218–24.

31. Martin RH. Sperm chromosome analysis in a man heterozygous for a paracentric inversion of chromosome 14 (q24.1q32.1). *Am J Hum Genet.* 1999;64:1480–4.

32. Bhatt S et al. Breakpoint mapping and complete analysis of meiotic segregation patterns in three men heterozygous for paracentric inversions. *Eur J Hum Genet.* Jan 2009;17(1):44–50.

33. Yapan C et al. The largest paracentric inversion, the highest rate of recombinant spermatozoa. Case Report: 46,XY,inv(2)(q21.2q37.3) and literature review. *Balkan J Med Genet.* 2014;17(1):55–62.

34. Morel F et al. Meiotic segregation analysis in spermatozoa of pericentric inversion carriers using fluorescence in-situ hybridization. *Hum Reprod.* Jan 2007;22(1):136–41.

35. Abdi A et al. Prevalence of chromosome inversions (pericentric and paracentric) in patients with recurrent abortions. *SJRM*. 2018;2(2):45–50.

36. Sharony R et al. Prenatal diagnosis of pericentric inversion in homologues of chromosome 9: A decision dilemma. *Am J Perinatol*. Feb 2007;24(2):137–40.

37. Anton E et al. Sperm studies in heterozygote inversion carriers: A review. *Cytogenet Genome Res*. 2005;111(3–4):297–304.

38. Scriven PN et al. Meiotic outcomes of three-way translocations ascertained in cleavage-stage embryos: Refinement of reproductive risks and implications for PGD. *Eur J Hum Genet*. 2014;22(6):748–53.

39. Salaun G et al. Sperm meiotic segregation of a balanced interchromosomal reciprocal insertion resulting in recurrent spontaneous miscarriage. *Reprod Biomed Online*. Jul 2018;37(1):100–6.

40. Melotte C et al. Preimplantation genetic diagnosis for an insertional translocation carrier. *Hum Reprod*. Dec 2004;19(12):2777–83.

41. Xanthopoulou L et al. Male and female meiotic behaviour of an intrachromosomal insertion determined by preimplantation genetic diagnosis. *Mol Cytogenet*. 2010;3(1):2.

42. Vanneste E et al. PGD for a complex chromosomal rearrangement by array comparative genomic hybridization. *Hum Reprod*. Apr 2011;26(4):941–9.

43. Pujol A et al. Multiple aneuploidies in the oocytes of balanced translocation carriers: A preimplantation genetic diagnosis study using first polar body. *Reproduction*. Dec 2003;126(6):701–11.

44. Molina Gomes D et al. Preconceptional diagnosis for Robertsonian translocation as an alternative to preimplantation genetic diagnosis in two situations: A pilot study. *J Assist Reprod Genet*. Mar 2009;26 (2–3):113–7.

45. Scott RT Jr et al. Cleavage-stage biopsy significantly impairs human embryonic implantation potential while blastocyst biopsy does not: A randomized and paired clinical trial. *Fertil Steril*. Sep 2013;100(3):624–30.

46. Gianaroli L et al. Blastocentesis: A source of DNA for preimplantation genetic testing. Results from a pilot study. *Fertil Steril*. Dec 2014;102(6):1692–9.e6.

47. Magli MC et al. Preimplantation genetic testing: Polar bodies, blastomeres, trophectoderm cells, or blastocoelic fluid? *Fertil Steril*. Mar 2016;105(3):676–83.

48. Liu W et al. Non-invasive pre-implantation aneuploidy screening and diagnosis of beta thalassemia IVSII654 mutation using spent embryo culture medium. *Ann Med*. Jun 2017;49(4):319–28.

49. Xu J et al. Noninvasive chromosome screening of human embryos by genome sequencing of embryo culture medium for in vitro fertilization. *Proc Natl Acad Sci U S A*. 18 Oct, 2016;113(42):11907–12.

50. Jiao J et al. Minimally invasive preimplantation genetic testing using blastocyst culture medium. *Hum Reprod*. 8 Jul, 2019;34(7):1369–79.

51. Griffin DK et al. Fluorescent in-situ hybridization to interphase nuclei of human preimplantation embryos with X and Y chromosome specific probes. *Hum Reprod*. Jan 1991;6(1):101–5.

52. Schrurs BM, Winston RM, Handyside AH. Preimplantation diagnosis of aneuploidy using fluorescent in-situ hybridization: Evaluation using a chromosome 18-specific probe. *Hum Reprod*. Feb 1993;8(2):296–301.

53. Cassel MJ et al. Carrier-specific breakpoint-spanning DNA probes: An approach to preimplantation genetic diagnosis in interphase cells. *Hum Reprod*. Sep 1997;12(9):2019–27.

54. Munné S et al. Outcome of preimplantation genetic diagnosis of translocations. *Fertil Steril*. Jun 2000;73(6):1209–18.

55. Munné S et al. Negligible interchromosomal effect in embryos of Robertsonian translocation carriers. *Reprod Biomed Online*. Mar 2005;10(3):363–9.

56. Velilla E, Escudero T, Munné S. Blastomere fixation techniques and risk of misdiagnosis for preimplantation genetic diagnosis of aneuploidy. *Reprod Biomed Online*. May–Jun 2002;4(3):210–7.

57. Ghevaria H et al. The origin and significance of additional aneuploidy events in couples undergoing preimplantation genetic diagnosis for translocations by array comparative genomic hybridization. *Reprod Biomed Online*. Feb 2016;32(2):178–89.

58. Verlinsky Y et al. Nuclear transfer for full karyotyping and preimplantation diagnosis for translocations. *Reprod Biomed Online*. Nov–Dec 2002;5(3):300–5.

59. Kuliev A et al. Conversion and non-conversion approach to preimplantation diagnosis for chromosomal rearrangements in 475 cycles. *Reprod Biomed Online*. Jul 2010;21(1):93–9.

60. Lim CK et al. Estimation of chromosomal imbalances in preimplantation embryos from preimplantation genetic diagnosis cycles of reciprocal translocations with or without acrocentric chromosomes. *Fertil Steril*. Dec 2008;90(6):2144–51.

61. Ko DS et al. Clinical outcomes of preimplantation genetic diagnosis (PGD) and analysis of meiotic segregation modes in reciprocal translocation carriers. *Am J Med Genet A*. Jun 2010;152A(6):1428–33.

62. Gianaroli L et al. Possible interchromosomal effect in embryos generated by gametes from translocation carriers. *Hum Reprod*. Dec 2002;17(12):3201–7.

63. Pujol A et al. The importance of aneuploidy screening in reciprocal translocation carriers. *Reproduction*. Jun 2006;131(6):1025–35.

64. Keymolen K et al. Preimplantation genetic diagnosis in female and male carriers of reciprocal translocations: Clinical outcome until delivery of 312 cycles. *Eur J Hum Genet*. Apr 2012;20(4):376–80.

65. Verlinsky Y et al. Preimplantation testing for chromosomal disorders improves reproductive outcome of poor-prognosis patients. *Reprod Biomed Online*. Aug 2005;11(2):219–25.

66. Franssen MT et al. Reproductive outcome after PGD in couples with recurrent miscarriage carrying a structural chromosome abnormality: A systematic review. *Hum Reprod Update*. Jul–Aug 2011;17(4):467–75.

67. Iews M et al. Does preimplantation genetic diagnosis improve reproductive outcome in couples with recurrent pregnancy loss owing to structural chromosomal rearrangement? A systematic review. *Reprod Biomed Online*. Jun 2018;36(6):677–85.

68. Traversa MV, Carey L, Leigh D. A molecular strategy for routine preimplantation genetic diagnosis in both reciprocal and Robertsonian translocation carriers. *Mol Hum Reprod*. May 2010;16(5):329–37.

69. Fiorentino F et al. Polymerase chain reaction-based detection of chromosomal imbalances on embryos: The evolution of preimplantation genetic diagnosis for chromosomal translocations. *Fertil Steril*. Nov 2010;94(6):2001–11, 2011.e1–6.

70. Malmgren H et al. Single cell CGH analysis reveals a high degree of mosaicism in human embryos from patients with balanced structural chromosome aberrations. *Mol Hum Reprod*. May 2002;8(5):502–10.

71. Le Caignec C et al. Single-cell chromosomal imbalances detection by array CGH. *Nucleic Acids Res*. 12 May, 2006;34(9):e68.

72. Kallioniemi A et al. Comparative genomic hybridization for molecular cytogenetic analysis of solid tumors. *Science*. 30 Oct, 1992;258(5083):818–21.

73. Wilton L. Preimplantation genetic diagnosis and chromosome analysis of blastomeres using comparative genomic hybridization. *Hum Reprod Update*. Jan–Feb 2005;11(1):33–41.

74. Rius M et al. Detection of unbalanced chromosome segregations in preimplantation genetic diagnosis of translocations by short comparative genomic hybridization. *Fertil Steril*. Jul 2011;96(1):134–42.

75. Hellani A et al. Successful pregnancies after application of array-comparative genomic hybridization in PGS-aneuploidy screening. *Reprod Biomed Online*. Dec 2008;17(6):841–7.

76. Fiorentino F et al. PGD for reciprocal and Robertsonian translocations using array comparative genomic hybridization. *Hum Reprod*. Jul 2011;26(7):1925–35.

77. Ramos L et al. Oligonucleotide arrays vs. metaphase-comparative genomic hybridization and BAC arrays for single-cell analysis: First applications to preimplantation genetic diagnosis for Robertsonian translocation carriers. *PLOS ONE*. 21 Nov, 2014;9(11):e113223.

78. Munné S. Preimplantation genetic diagnosis for aneuploidy and translocations using array comparative genomic hybridization. *Curr Genomics*. Sep 2012;13(6):463–70.

79. Colls P et al. Validation of array comparative genome hybridization for diagnosis of translocations in preimplantation human embryos. *Reprod Biomed Online*. Jun 2012;24(6):621–9.

80. Christodoulou C et al. Preimplantation genetic diagnosis for chromosomal rearrangements with the use of array comparative genomic hybridization at the blastocyst stage. *Fertil Steril*. Jan 2017;107(1):212–9.e3.

81. Alfarawati S et al. First births after preimplantation genetic diagnosis of structural chromosome abnormalities using comparative genomic hybridization and microarray analysis. *Hum Reprod*. Jun 2011;26(6):1560–74.

82. Handyside AH et al. Karyomapping: A universal method for genome wide analysis of genetic disease based on mapping crossovers between parental haplotypes. *J Med Genet*. Oct 2010;47(10):651–8.

83. Treff NR et al. Accurate single cell 24 chromosome aneuploidy screening using whole genome amplification and single nucleotide polymorphism microarrays. *Fertil Steril*. Nov 2010;94(6):2017–21.

84. Treff NR et al. Single nucleotide polymorphism microarray-based concurrent screening of 24-chromosome aneuploidy and unbalanced translocations in preimplantation human embryos. *Fertil Steril.* Apr 2011a;95(5):1606–12.e1–2.

85. Treff NR et al. Use of single nucleotide polymorphism microarrays to distinguish between balanced and normal chromosomes in embryos from a translocation carrier. *Fertil Steril.* Jul 2011b;96(1):e58–65.

86. Treff NR et al. SNP array-based analyses of unbalanced embryos as a reference to distinguish between balanced translocation carrier and normal blastocysts. *J Assist Reprod Genet.* Aug 2016;33(8):1115–9.

87. Sundheimer LW et al. Diagnosis of parental balanced reciprocal translocations by trophectoderm biopsy and comprehensive chromosomal screening. *J Assist Reprod Genet.* Jan 2018;35(1):165–9.

88. Zhang S et al. The establishment and application of preimplantation genetic haplotyping in embryo diagnosis for reciprocal and Robertsonian translocation carriers. *BMC Med Genomics.* 17 Oct, 2017;10(1):60.

89. Zhang S et al. BasePhasing: A highly efficient approach for preimplantation genetic haplotyping in clinical application of balanced translocation carriers. *BMC Med Genomics.* 18 Mar, 2019;12(1):52.

90. van Uum CM et al. SNP array-based copy number and genotype analyses for preimplantation genetic diagnosis of human unbalanced translocations. *Eur J Hum Genet.* Sep 2012;20(9):938–44.

91. Tan YQ et al. Single-nucleotide polymorphism microarray-based preimplantation genetic diagnosis is likely to improve the clinical outcome for translocation carriers. *Hum Reprod.* Sep 2013;28(9):2581–92.

92. Tobler KJ et al. Two different microarray technologies for preimplantation genetic diagnosis and screening, due to reciprocal translocation imbalances, demonstrate equivalent euploidy and clinical pregnancy rates. *J Assist Reprod Genet.* Jul 2014;31(7):843–50.

93. Xiong B et al. Using SNP array to identify aneuploidy and segmental imbalance in translocation carriers. *Genom Data.* 24 May, 2014;2:92–5.

94. Idowu D et al. Pregnancy outcomes following 24-chromosome preimplantation genetic diagnosis in couples with balanced reciprocal or Robertsonian translocations. *Fertil Steril.* Apr 2015;103(4):1037–42.

95. Wang YZ et al. Number of blastocysts biopsied as a predictive indicator to obtain at least one normal/ balanced embryo following preimplantation genetic diagnosis with single nucleotide polymorphism microarray in translocation cases. *J Assist Reprod Genet.* Jan 2017;34(1):51–9.

96. Kubicek D et al. Incidence and origin of meiotic whole and segmental chromosomal aneuploidies detected by karyomapping. *Reprod Biomed Online.* Mar 2019;38(3):330–9.

97. Beyer CE et al. Preimplantation genetic testing using Karyomapping for a paternally inherited reciprocal translocation: A case study. *J Assist Reprod Genet.* May 2019;36(5):951–63.

98. Knapp M, Stiller M, Meyer M. Generating barcoded libraries for multiplex high-throughput sequencing. *Methods Mol Biol.* 2012;840:155–70.

99. Wells D et al. Clinical utilisation of a rapid low-pass whole genome sequencing technique for the diagnosis of aneuploidy in human embryos prior to implantation. *J Med Genet.* Aug 2014;51(8):553–62.

100. Maxwell SM et al. Why do euploid embryos miscarry? A case-control study comparing the rate of aneuploidy within presumed euploid embryos that resulted in miscarriage or live birth using next-generation sequencing. *Fertil Steril.* Nov 2016;106(6):1414–9.e5.

101. Morin SJ et al. Translocations, inversions and other chromosome rearrangements. *Fertil Steril.* Jan 2017;107(1):19–26.

102. Bono S et al. Validation of a semiconductor next-generation sequencing-based protocol for preimplantation genetic diagnosis of reciprocal translocations. *Prenat Diagn.* Oct 2015;35(10):938–44.

103. Cuman C et al. Defining the limits of detection for chromosome rearrangements in the preimplantation embryo using next generation sequencing. *Hum Reprod.* 2018;33(8): 1566–76.

104. Yin X et al. Massively parallel sequencing for chromosomal abnormality testing in trophectoderm cells of human blastocysts. *Biol Reprod.* 21 Mar, 2013;88(3):69.

105. Tan Y et al. Clinical outcome of preimplantation genetic diagnosis and screening using next generation sequencing. *Gigascience.* 4 Dec, 2014;3(1):30.

106. Gui B et al. Chromosomal analysis of blastocysts from balanced chromosomal rearrangement carriers. *Reproduction.* Apr 2016;151(4):455–64.

107. Chow JFC et al. Evaluation of preimplantation genetic testing for chromosomal structural rearrangement by a commonly used next generation sequencing workflow. *Eur J Obstet Gynecol Reprod Biol.* May 2018;224:66–73.

108. Zhang W et al. Clinical application of next-generation sequencing in preimplantation genetic diagnosis cycles for Robertsonian and reciprocal translocations. *J Assist Reprod Genet.* Jul 2016;33(7):899–906.

109. Wang J et al. Analysis of meiotic segregation modes in biopsied blastocysts from preimplantation genetic testing cycles of reciprocal translocations. *Mol Cytogenet.* 26 Feb, 2019;12:11.

110. Wang L et al. Preferential selection and transfer of euploid noncarrier embryos in preimplantation genetic diagnosis cycles for reciprocal translocations. *Fertil Steril.* Oct 2017;108(4):620–7.e4.

111. Lledó B et al. The paternal effect of chromosome translocation carriers observed from meiotic segregation in embryos. *Hum Reprod.* Jul 2010;25(7):1843–8.

112. Ye Y et al. Meiotic segregation analysis of embryos from reciprocal translocation carriers in PGD cycles. *Reprod Biomed Online.* Jan 2012;24(1):83–90.

113. Chang EM et al. Preimplantation genetic diagnosis for couples with a Robertsonian translocation: Practical information for genetic counseling. *J Assist Reprod Genet.* Jan 2012;29(1):67–75.

114. Zhang L et al. Effects of a carrier's sex and age on the segregation patterns of the trivalent of Robertsonian translocations. *J Assist Reprod Genet.* Sep 2019;36(9):1963–9.

115. Zhang L et al. Interaction of acrocentric chromosome involved in translocation and sex of the carrier influences the proportion of alternate segregation in autosomal reciprocal translocations. *Hum Reprod.* 1 Feb, 2019;34(2):380–7.

116. LeMaire-Adkins R, Radke K, Hunt PA. Lack of checkpoint control at the metaphase/anaphase transition: A mechanism of meiotic nondisjunction in mammalian females. *J Cell Biol.* 29 Dec, 1997;139(7):1611–9.

117. Xie Y et al. Preliminary analysis of numerical chromosome abnormalities in reciprocal and Robertsonian translocation preimplantation genetic diagnosis cases with 24-chromosomal analysis with an aCGH/SNP microarray. *J Assist Reprod Genet.* Jan 2018;35(1):177–86.

118. Lejeune J. Autosomal disorders. *Pediatrics.* Sep 1963;32:326–37.

119. Lindenbaum RH et al. The prevalence of translocations in parents of children with regular trisomy 21: A possible interchromosomal effect? *J Med Genet.* Feb 1985;22(1):24–8.

120. Navarro J et al. XY-trivalent association and synaptic anomalies in a male carrier of a Robertsonian t(13;14) translocation. *Hum Reprod.* Mar 1991;6(3):376–81.

121. Solé M et al. Altered bivalent positioning in metaphase I human spermatocytes from Robertsonian translocation carriers. *J Assist Reprod Genet.* Jan 2017;34(1):131–8.

122. Pellestor F et al. Study of the occurrence of interchromosomal effect in spermatozoa of chromosomal rearrangement carriers by fluorescence in-situ hybridization and primed in-situ labelling techniques. *Hum Reprod.* Jun 2001;16(6):1155–64.

123. Godo A et al. Accumulation of numerical and structural chromosome imbalances in spermatozoa from reciprocal translocation carriers. *Hum Reprod.* Mar 2013;28(3):840–9.

124. Scriven PN et al. Robertsonian translocations-reproductive risks and indications for preimplantation genetic diagnosis. *Hum Reprod.* Nov 2001;16(11):2267–73.

125. Munné S. Analysis of chromosome segregation during preimplantation genetic diagnosis in both male and female translocation heterozygotes. *Cytogenet Genome Res.* 2005;111(3–4):305–9.

126. Hamerton JL et al. A cytogenetic survey of 14,069 newborn infants. I. Incidence of chromosome abnormalities. *Clin Genet.* Oct 1975;8(4):223–43.

127. Ferfouri F et al. Can one translocation impact the meiotic segregation of another translocation? A sperm-FISH analysis of a 46,XY,t(1;16)(q21;p11.2),t(8;9)(q24.3;p24) patient and his 46,XY,t(8;9)(q24.3;p24) brother and cousin. *Mol Hum Reprod.* Feb 2013;19(2):109–17.

128. Young D et al. Infertility patients with chromosome inversions are not susceptible to an inter-chromosomal effect. *J Assist Reprod Genet.* Mar 2019;36(3):509–16.

129. Vanneste E et al. What next for preimplantation genetic screening? High mitotic chromosome instability rate provides the biological basis for the low success rate. *Hum Reprod.* Nov 2009;24(11):2679–82.

130. Alfarawati S et al. Embryos of Robertsonian translocation carriers exhibit a mitotic interchromosomal effect that enhances genetic instability during early development. *PLOS GENET.* 2012;8(10):e1003025.

131. Benkhalifa M et al. Cytogenetics of uncleaved oocytes and arrested zygotes in IVF programs. *J Assist Reprod Genet.* Feb 1996;13(2):140–8.

132. Findikli N et al. Assessment of DNA fragmentation and aneuploidy on poor quality human embryos. *Reprod Biomed Online.* Feb 2004;8(2):196–206.

133. Evsikov S, Cieslak J, Verlinsky Y. Effect of chromosomal translocations on the development of preimplantation human embryos in vitro. *Fertil Steril.* Oct 2000;74(4):672–7.

134. Findikli N et al. Embryo development characteristics in Robertsonian and reciprocal translocations: A comparison of results with non-translocation cases. *Reprod Biomed Online*. Nov 2003;7(5):563–71.

135. Campbell A et al. Modelling a risk classification of aneuploidy in human embryos using non-invasive morphokinetics. *Reprod Biomed Online*. May 2013;26(5):477–85.

136. Meseguer M et al. The use of morphokinetics as a predictor of embryo implantation. *Hum Reprod*. 2011 Oct;26(10):2658–71.

137. Jones CA et al. PGD for a carrier of an intrachromosomal insertion using aCGH. *Syst Biol Reprod Med*. Dec 2014;60(6):377–82.

138. Amir H et al. Time-lapse imaging reveals delayed development of embryos carrying unbalanced chromosomal translocations. *J Assist Reprod Genet*. Feb 2019;36(2):315–24.

139. Lammers J et al. Morphokinetic parameters in chromosomal translocation carriers undergoing preimplantation genetic testing. *Reprod Biomed Online*. Feb 2019;38(2):177–83.

140. Chen SH et al. Patterns of ovarian response to gonadotropin stimulation in female carriers of balanced translocation. *Fertil Steril*. May 2005;83(5):1504–9.

141. Dechanet C et al. Do female translocations influence the ovarian response pattern to controlled ovarian stimulation in preimplantation genetic diagnosis? *Hum Reprod*. May 2011;26(5):1232–40.

142. Chen W et al. Breakpoint analysis of balanced chromosome rearrangements by next-generation paired-end sequencing. *Eur J Hum Genet*. May 2010;18(5):539–43.

143. Wu T et al. First report on an X-linked hypohidrotic ectodermal dysplasia family with X chromosome inversion: Breakpoint mapping reveals the pathogenic mechanism and preimplantation genetics diagnosis achieves an unaffected birth. *Clin Chim Acta*. Dec 2017;475:78–84.

144. Krantz ID et al. Deletions of 20p12 in Alagille syndrome: Frequency and molecular characterization. *Am J Med Genet*. 2 May, 1997;70(1):80–6.

145. Hu L et al. Reciprocal translocation carrier diagnosis in preimplantation human embryos. *EBioMedicine* Dec 2016;14:139–47.

146. Machev N et al. Fluorescence in situ hybridization sperm analysis of six translocation carriers provides evidence of an interchromosomal effect. *Fertil Steril*. Aug 2005;84(2):365–73.

147. Pellestor F et al. Complex chromosomal rearrangements: Origin and meiotic behavior. *Hum Reprod Update*. Jul–Aug 2011;17(4):476–94.

148. Hu L et al. Clinical outcomes in carriers of complex chromosomal rearrangements: A retrospective analysis of comprehensive chromosome screening results in seven cases. *Fertil Steril*. Mar 2018;109(3):486–92.

5

Preimplantation Genetic Testing for Monogenic Disorders

Martine De Rycke and Pieter Verdyck

CONTENTS

Introduction

The previous terms preimplantation genetic diagnosis (PGD) and preimplantation genetic screening (PGS) have been replaced by the term preimplantation genetic testing (PGT), following a revision of terminology used in infertility care [1]. PGT can be performed for aneuploidy detection (PGT-A), for monogenic disorders or single-gene defects (PGT-M) and for chromosomal structural rearrangements (PGT-SR). PGT involves the biopsy of a single or few cells from *in vitro* fertilized oocytes (polar bodies) or embryos (cleavage stage or blastocyst) and testing of the biopsied cell(s) for genetic abnormalities or for human leukocyte antigen (HLA) typing. The selective transfer of embryos unaffected for the condition under study circumvents invasive prenatal diagnosis and possible therapeutic termination of pregnancy. PGT requires an *in vitro* fertilization (IVF) treatment; this treatment, with additional risks and costs, may be considered a burden for fertile couples. Couples at risk of transmitting a genetic condition and concurrently suffering from infertility may more easily combine IVF and PGT.

Although genetic testing of single cells is challenging and the overall procedure is quite complex, PGT has evolved from an experimental procedure into a well-established alternative to invasive prenatal diagnosis. The first report on children born after PGT was by Handyside et al. in 1990, describing the use of polymerase chain reaction (PCR) for the detection of repetitive Y-sequences for gender determination in families with X-linked diseases [2]. Simplex PCR was replaced by single-cell multiplex PCR, which became the method of choice for the detection of monogenic disorders. Genome-wide technologies began to replace the gold standard method of PCR over the last decade, in parallel with a shift in biopsy stage from a single blastomere biopsied at day 3 to 5–10 trophectoderm (TE) cells biopsied at day 5/6. This allowed for concurrent analysis of PGT-M together with PGT-A, the latter aiming at increasing pregnancy rates and decreasing miscarriage rate per embryo transfer.

Indications

PGT-M is available for (combinations of) monogenic disorders for which the disease-causing loci have been unequivocally identified. These loci are nuclear (X-linked, autosomal dominantly, or recessively inherited) or mitochondrial (maternally inherited) and involve (likely) pathogenic germline genetic variant(s) (class 4–5) [3]. Molecular genetic reports stating the disease-causing mutation(s) are mandatory at the intake of a PGT request. The more frequently occurring disorders for which PGT-M is currently applied are cystic fibrosis for the autosomal recessive disorders, and myotonic dystrophy type 1, neurofibromatosis, Huntington disease, and hereditary breast and ovarian cancer (*BRCA1/BRCA2* mutations) for the autosomal dominant disorders. For the X-linked disorders, PGT is mainly carried out for Duchenne muscular dystrophy, hemophilia, and fragile X syndrome. The advantages of specific DNA diagnosis over sexing for X-linked disorders are twofold: healthy male embryos are not discarded, and female carrier embryos can be identified and possibly used for transfer, according to the patient's wishes and the center's policy.

PGT was initially applied for the same indications as in prenatal diagnosis. Later, the list of indications also started to include indications for which prenatal diagnosis is regarded as ethically difficult, such as late-onset disorders and cancer predisposition syndromes with incomplete penetrance [4]. The use of PGT is legally restricted in many countries; however, policies and regulations differ. In some countries the law is quite restrictive with a clear line between acceptable and unacceptable indications, while in other countries the law is more liberal without specific mechanisms in place for delineating which indications are eligible for PGT. Some special indications have raised further ethical concerns.

Human leukocyte antigen (HLA) matching of preimplantation embryos is an exceptional indication as it is not a pathologic condition. The aim is to select an embryo that is HLA-compatible with an affected sibling. Hematopoietic stem cells from the cord blood at birth or later from bone marrow of the savior baby are used to transplant and cure the affected sibling. HLA typing alone is carried out for acquired diseases related to the hematopoietic and/or immune system, such as leukemias. Alternatively, HLA typing is combined with the detection of mutations underlying single-gene disorders, mostly immunodeficiencies and hemoglobinopathies [5,6]. The selection of HLA-matched embryos has evoked many ethical debates. The possible instrumentalization of the child to be born is the main issue raised in these discussions. As a result, the regulation of PGT and HLA matching varies in different countries around the world. Local and national legislation usually allow the use of PGT to avoid the transmission of diseases for which no treatment exists, but only a subset of frameworks is permissive for PGT and HLA typing, and often extra conditions apply. For instance, the Belgian law stipulates that within every PGT request for HLA matching the motives of the couple must be evaluated.

PGT and HLA matching should only be considered when all other clinical options have been exhausted (i.e., no suitable matched related donors are available, or no suitable unrelated donors can be obtained from registries). The genetic chance of finding an embryo HLA-matched to the affected sibling is only 25%. The genetic selection in cases of HLA matching along with excluding a monogenic disease is even more stringent, with theoretical chances of 19% for autosomal recessive disorders or 12.5% for autosomal dominant or X-linked disorders. The gold standard for HLA typing of preimplantation embryos is an indirect test with genetic markers across the region. The large size of the region and the inherent high recombination frequency impose technical limitations. Another constraint is female age, as women opting for PGT with HLA matching are often of advanced maternal age, and female age is one of the strongest negative predictors for a successful outcome. When combining all the aforementioned limitations, it is clear that the overall success rate of PGT and HLA matching is lower than the general PGT-M outcome. Furthermore, consideration should be given to the time required for preclinical workup, cycle(s) application, and for an HLA-matched sibling to be born, implying that PGT with HLA matching may be a valuable option when the affected child does not need immediate medical intervention.

In families with a history of late-onset diseases such as Huntington disease, individuals at risk who want to avoid presymptomatic testing but wish for their own biological children to be free of the disease may opt for PGT with exclusion testing [7]. Such testing is indirect and involves the transfer of embryos carrying the haplotype derived from the non-affected grandparent. Embryos that have inherited the haplotype of the affected grandparent will be discarded, as they have a 50% chance of being affected. These embryos also have a 50% chance of being healthy for the disease under study. This fact, together with the fact that about half of the couples will have an unnecessary IVF/PGT treatment with exposure to side effects and risks for the female and embryo, may be considered unethical. PGT with exclusion testing is therefore prohibited in some countries. The alternative, with direct testing and nondisclosure of the results, is not recommended as it obligates extreme confidentiality and causes further moral and ethical issues.

The majority of mitochondrial DNA (mtDNA) mutations implicated in diseases show heteroplasmy, which is the coexistence of wild-type and mutant mtDNA in a single cell. The mtDNA mutation load (proportion of mutant mtDNA) may vary over time and differ from one cell type to another. Clinical symptoms are displayed once a particular mutation load threshold has been exceeded. Because of a genetic bottleneck during oogenesis, the proportion of mutant mtDNA inherited from one generation to the next varies widely. PGT can be applied to select embryos with zero or low mtDNA mutation load, with the latter option reducing the risk for an affected child rather than eliminating it [8]. Mutation load analysis via PCR followed by restriction fragment length polymorphism or via next-generation sequencing (NGS) is technically accurate [9]. The difficulties lie in the many unknowns associated with risk estimation and establishing a mutation-specific threshold below which embryo transfer is acceptable. It has been established for the more common mtDNA mutations that the mutation load of a blastomere from cleavage stage is predictive of the entire embryo, but it remains unclear whether this can be extrapolated to all mtDNA mutations and to biopsied samples from blastocysts [10,11]. For rare mutations, it is warranted to assess the variation in mutation load within embryos (for instance in arrested embryos of the first cycle). Prenatal diagnosis as well as follow-up of the children is indicated to verify whether mutation load is consistent with the mutation load observed in the embryos. For carriers of homoplasmic mutant mtDNA or carriers producing only embryos with high mutation loads, PGT is not a suitable option. As a consequence of the high clinical and genetic complexity of mitochondrial disorders, few centers offer PGT and have gained experience on this topic. As more data become available, the general utility of PGT for this difficult group of disorders may expand.

As the procedure relies on the selection of embryos, PGT is not possible if the parents do not possess wild-type alleles, e.g., when both parents are affected with an autosomal recessive disorder or the female partner is homoplasmic for a mitochondrial mutation. For these indications, alternative technologies such as pronuclear or oocyte spindle transfer (for mitochondrial disorders) [12] and genome editing are being developed, which may prove to be valuable technologies in the future [13].

Diagnostic Methods

Multiplex Fluorescent PCR

Amplification methods are required to increase the limited amount of genomic DNA in the embryonic samples. Amplification is carried out following embryo biopsy: the single or multiple biopsied cells are washed, transferred to reaction tubes, and lysed. Amplification reaction components are then added directly to the lysed cell(s) without prior DNA purification. At the start of PGT for monogenic disorders in the early nineties, simplex PCR amplification for detection of the mutation was applied. If the mutation did not generate a difference in amplicon fragment length, digestion with appropriate restriction enzymes was applied to allow differentiation of wild-type and mutant alleles. From these earliest approaches, contamination and allele dropout (ADO) soon surfaced as two important issues that could lead to misdiagnosis. Contamination with extraneous DNA or carryover from previous amplification reactions is a major problem, given the high number of amplification cycles that is required to increase the minute amount of DNA. ADO derives from the unequal amplification of alleles present in a heterozygous sample (called preferential amplification) to the point where an allele remains undetected. High working standards and rigorous prevention measures were used to prevent and control for contamination. ADO, on the other hand, was minimized by using well-optimized methods for cell lysis and amplification and the use of the most sensitive methods for allele detection (for instance, fluorescently labeled primers). The most important measure, however, was the addition of primers for closely linked informative short-tandem repeat (STR) markers to the amplification mix. With every added informative marker, the diagnosis is confirmed and contamination and ADO for an individual marker or mutation amplicon can be detected, thereby increasing the accuracy of the test. The development of a well-equilibrated duplex or triplex test was often cumbersome in the early days. Often, amplification products from a duplex or triplex PCR reaction with 10 to 20 cycles were used as a template for a second round of simplex PCR (often with nested or semi-nested primers) if the amplicons were incompatible. Fortunately, the process of multiplexing was facilitated with the availability of commercial PCR multiplex kits, now allowing multiplexing of over a dozen amplicons.

In practice, PGT-M with multiplex PCR can be subdivided in informativity testing, multiplex PCR optimization, and the actual clinical PGT cycle. For informativity testing, DNA and genetic reports from the couple and relevant family members are collected. STR markers located close to the gene of interest are genotyped to allow for selection of informative STR markers that flank the gene of interest. Preferably, the selected STR markers allow discrimination of all parental haplotypes. The haplotype that is shared between the relatives carrying the familial mutation is then inferred as the risk haplotype. If the risk haplotype is determined during workup, an indirect strategy can be chosen using STR markers only for the clinical PGT cycle. Alternatively, a direct strategy is possible where the detection of the mutation(s) is added to the STR markers for confirmation of phasing [14].

The optimization of a new multiplex PCR test is labor intensive. Hereto amplicons are equilibrated at the single-cell level and then validated on a large series of single cells. Lymphocytes, lymphoblasts, fibroblasts, or buccal cells are used as cell models during validation. As these steps of single-cell adaptation and validation have to be repeated for every new DNA locus, it represents a major bottleneck for targeted PCR-based methods.

For some couples it is not possible to determine on which STR marker haplotype the mutation is located—for example, when a *de novo* mutation is present in one of the partners or when no relevant family DNA samples can be obtained. In these special cases, phase may be determined and diagnosis can be obtained during the first PGT cycle when using a direct strategy and on conditions that sufficient embryos are available, that at least one embryo is diagnosed as affected, and the mutation is consistently detected in the presence of the same parental haplotype. As targeted PCR-based amplification is mostly coupled with day 3 biopsy, the number of (affected) embryos is usually adequate to support phasing.

Many types of mutations can be detected by PCR supplemented with a post-PCR reaction if necessary. Deletion or duplication mutations of a few nucleotides can be detected directly via detection of fragment length difference. For single-nucleotide substitutions, different strategies of PCR and allele discrimination have been developed, such as amplification refractory mutation system [15], endonuclease restriction [15], Sanger sequencing or mini-sequencing [16], and quantitative real-time PCR [17]. Direct detection of complex and/or larger gene rearrangements is often not feasible, as the exact breakpoints of the rearrangement are frequently unknown. An example of informativity testing (a) and clinical PGT results (b) carried out via an indirect targeted multiplex PCR are shown in Figure 5.1.

High diagnostic accuracy and efficiency were achieved with multiplex fluorescent PCR, and this approach was the gold standard for over two decades. However, as the optimization of customized multiplex PCR tests is very labor intensive, this stimulated the development of more generic approaches. The method of PCR-based haplotyping with prior single- or few-cell whole-genome amplification (WGA) followed by standard PCR reactions of a multitude of STRs flanking the region(s) of interest is already a more general method than targeted single-cell PCR because the adaptation/validation of PCR reactions to the single-cell level can be omitted [18]. The implementation of WGA followed by single nucleotide polymorphism (SNP) array represents a shift toward truly generic methods.

Whole-Genome Amplification

WGA overcomes the problem of the minute quantity of gDNA by amplifying the entire genome of single or few cells up to several micrograms, which proves sufficient template for several standard downstream applications. This represents a major technical improvement, which together with the shift from cleavage-stage to blastocyst biopsy and the introduction of more successful embryo cryopreservation methods has revolutionized the field of PGT, offering a range of robust testing strategies.

(a)

Indication	OMIM disease	Inheritance	Gene	OMIM gene	Ref Seq	Mat mutation	Pat mutation
Charcot-Marie-Tooth disease, type 1A	118220	AD	PMP22	601097	NM_0003042	gene duplication	/

Informativity results

Locus	Location relative to gene	Informativity	Family members			
			aff female	male	father of female	aff mother
Amelogenin			116-116	116-121	116-116	116-121
PMP22						
D17S2230	210 Kb 5'	Informative	268-(278-294)*	257-288	263-268	294-(278-294)*
D17S122	41 Kb 5'	Informative	216-(214-216)*	206-214	208-216	216-(214-216)*
PMP22str23AC	15 Kb 3'	Informative	164-(152-164)*	162-162	152-164	152-(152-164)*
D17S2229	74 Kb 3'	Not Informative	231-(231-231)*	225-233	239-231	241-(231-231)*
D17S2227	517 Kb 3'	Informative	177-(152-167)*	162-157	157-177	152-(152-167)*
D17S2220	790 Kb 3'	Informative	316-(322-323)*	314-318	297-316	310-(322-323)*

(b)

aff female	male	Locus	Relative location	Tubing	E1.1	E3.1	E5.1	E6.1	E7.1	E8.1	E10.1	E11.1
				OK	OK	OK	OK	OK	OK	OK	OK	OK
PMP22												
268-(278-294)*	257-288	D17S2230 FAM	210 Kb 5'		268-257	268-257	268-288	(278-294)*-288	268-257	(278-294)*-288	(278-294)*-288	268-257
216-(214-216)*	206-214	D17S1220TN HEX	41 Kb 5'		216-206	216-206	216-214	(214-216)*-214	216-206	(214-216)*-214	(214-216)*-214	216-206
164-(152-164)*	162-162	PMP22str23AC NED	15 Kb 3'		164-162	164-162	164-162	(152-164)*-162	164-162	(152-164)*-162	(152-164)*-162	164-162
231-(231-231)*	225-233	D17S2229 NED	74 Kb 3'		231-225	231-225	231-233	(231-231)*-233	231-225	(231-231)*-233	(231-231)*-233	231-225
177-(152-167)*	162-157	D17S2227 FAM	517 Kb 3'		177-162	177-162	177-157	(152-167)*-157	177-162	(152-167)*-157	(152-167)*-157	177-162
316-(322-323)*	314-318	D17S2220 HEX	790 Kb 3'		316-314	316-314?	316-318	(322-323)*-318	316-314	(322-323)*-318	(322-323)*-318	316-314
Negative Control Intern: OK			Blanks	ok	ok	ok	ok	OK	OK	OK	OK	OK
Negative Control Extern:			Remarks									
			DIAGNOSIS CELL		Unaffected	Unaffected	Unaffected	Affected	Unaffected	Affected	Affected	Unaffected
			DIAGNOSIS EMBRYO		Unaffected	Unaffected	Unaffected	Affected	Unaffected	Affected	Affected	Unaffected

FIGURE 5.1 (a) Informativity testing and (b) clinical PGT results carried out via an indirect targeted multiplex PCR.

Many WGA protocols have been published over time and some of them are available as commercial kits. The first WGA methods were PCR-based and suffered from very incomplete genome coverage and amplification bias. The use of Taq DNA polymerase yielded an average fragment length of 400–500 bp (with a maximum size of 3 kb) and introduced many DNA sequence errors. A multiple displacement amplification (MDA) method relying on isothermal strand displacement amplification was established at the single-cell level more than a decade ago [19]. In an MDA reaction, random exonuclease-resistant primers anneal to the denatured target DNA and a DNA polymerase with strand-displacement activity such as Phi29 elongates the primers in an isothermal reaction at 30°C. Additional priming events can occur on each displaced strand leading to a network of branched DNA strands over 10 kb. Because of the proofreading activity of the Phi29 polymerase, the error rate of MDA-based WGA is much lower compared with Taq DNA polymerase–based methods, but the non-linear amplification yields over- or underrepresentation of genomic regions [20].

Later, WGA methods combining MDA and PCR amplification were introduced. Both the Rubicon PicoPLEX and the MALBAC (Multiple Annealing and Looping-Based Amplification Cycles) protocol initiate with DNA fragmentation and a preamplification MDA reaction using hybrid primers, followed by PCR [21,22].

None of the WGA methods are producing a true linear representation of the single- or few-cell genome and the results vary in ADO, preferential amplification rate, coverage, and nucleotide copy errors. As a consequence, a specific WGA method is chosen in function of the downstream application. The Rubicon PicoPLEX protocol is currently the method of choice for the detection of chromosomal copy number because of the reduced amplification bias, and MDA is preferred for haplotyping applications in cases of monogenic disorders because of better genome coverage and low error rates [23–25]. Final data interpretation has to take into account bias and artifacts introduced from WGA. Also, artifacts from cell-cycle phase should be considered. Analysis of TE samples with cells in different cell-cycle stages may overcome this problem, while the WGA representation bias may be partially filtered out by computational algorithms but cannot be completely eliminated.

SNP Array

Following WGA, either an approach of STR-based haplotyping via targeted PCR is applied, or WGA products are analyzed via a generic platform, SNP array, or NGS-based technology. SNP arrays are high-density oligo arrays containing up to several million probes, which allow genotyping of hundreds of thousands of selected SNPs across all chromosomes in a single reaction. SNPs are mostly biallelic, alleles are indicated as A and B, and genotypes are homozygous AA or BB, or heterozygous AB. The commercially available SNP arrays use different methods for SNP genotyping: hybridization to SNP allele–specific probes or single-base extension reactions are often applied [26]. The arrays are scanned, and SNP genotypes are called based on the total fluorescence and the ratio of hybridization intensities for A and B (allele frequencies) (e.g., AB is called in case of similar intensities of an intermediate level). Targeted multiplex PCR and SNP array share the same principle of linkage-based testing, but the SNP array workflow is much more standardized and uniform, without the need for a locus-specific preclinical workup. This reduces the laboratory workload and the waiting time for the couples substantially. Only a short family-specific workup with analysis of genomic DNA samples of the couple and a suitable reference (child or grandparent with known genetic status) is recommended to determine the number of informative SNPs in the region of interest and to establish phasing. The SNP array platform is especially powerful for double indications (for instance, two monogenic disorders or a monogenic disorder with HLA matching): following a minimal workup, whole-genome haplotyping is accomplished from a single data set. Haplotyping via SNP array can also be applied for balanced translocations or inversions: analysis reaches a high resolution and allows us to distinguish normal from balanced translocation carriers. The major requirements for SNP array application are that the chromosomal or monogenic aberration(s) are inherited, and relevant family samples are available for haplotyping. An example of a SNP array–based preclinical workup and clinical results for PGT-M are shown in Figure 5.2.

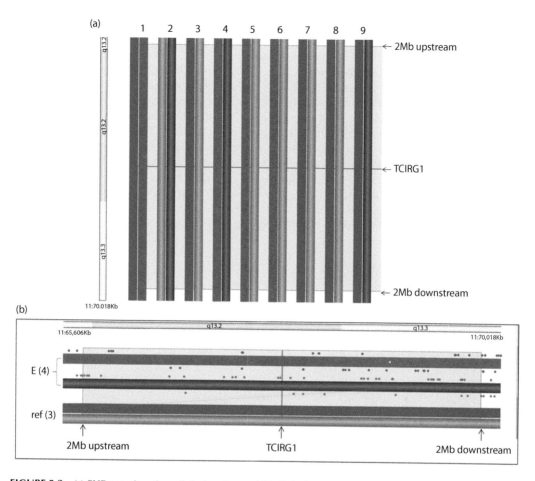

FIGURE 5.2 (a) SNP array-based preclinical workup and (b) clinical results for PGT-M.

Fresh embryo transfer is feasible with SNP array analysis and blastomere biopsy at day 3. The problem of limited time for analysis in the case of biopsy at day 5/6 is overcome by cryopreservation (relying on efficient vitrification and warming-survival protocols) and embryo transfer in a deferred cycle. This latter strategy enables a more efficient and cost-effective laboratory organization, as the larger time windows make it possible to pool and co-process samples of multiple patients.

Different SNP genotyping algorithms are available. Handyside and coworkers developed karyomapping, a family-based computational phasing approach for reconstruction of SNP haplotypes which flank the mutations [27,28]. It is applicable for both SNP arrays and NGS. Karyomapping uses discrete diploid SNP calls (assuming AA, BB, AB, or No call as possible states for each SNP) together with basic Mendelian laws, and requires a close relative for phasing. The karyomapping protocol has been commercially available since 2013 but the high costs of equipment and consumables seem to hamper its widespread clinical use. The fact that the underlying algorithm does not provide an all-in-one solution for concurrent molecular and chromosomal diagnosis may play a role as well.

PGT-M and PGT-A with SNPa

The use of PGT-A for specific IVF patient groups remains an ongoing debate, and there is no consensus about adding PGT-A routinely to PGT-M cases, yet concurrent PGT-A and PGT-M is increasingly regarded as an acceptable option since it does not entail additional procedures or higher risks for the couple or future child.

SNP array can allow for simultaneous analysis of PGT-M and PGT-A, as both SNP genotype and chromosome copy number info are obtained from the raw data set. As such, SNP arrays can reveal the presence of aneuploidies, polyploidies, and uniparental disomy. Two measures provide evidence about the copy number state: the log R ratio (the log2 transformed value of the normalized intensity of the SNP) and the B-allele frequency (BAF, which is the signal intensity of the B-allele over the total signal intensity for a SNP). BAF values of 0, 0.5, and 1 represent a normal copy number ($n = 2$) but aberrations will cause a decrease or increase of the total intensity and allele frequencies. SNP arrays at the level of a single or few cells yield a lot of noise because of WGA pitfalls, and therefore demand particularly well-developed algorithms for data interpretation. Genotyping algorithms using discrete diploid SNP calls such as karyomapping will yield errors across regions with copy number variations (true or WGA-induced) and therefore have restrictions in the detection of copy number aberrations. Some PGT centers rely on in-house-developed extended or novel algorithms to overcome this limitation. Haplarithmisis is a different computational pipeline; it primarily relies on continuous BAFs and allows haplotype and copy number detection as well as determination of the parental origin of the chromosomal anomaly [29].

Sequencing

NGS involves DNA fragmentation and preparation of a library of templates using adapters containing barcodes for a more affordable analysis with multiple samples in a single run. The single-molecule templates are then sequenced in parallel from one end or from both ends, either directly (third-generation) or after prior clonal amplification (second-generation), and the sequence reads are mapped to a reference genome. A crucial parameter is the genome coverage or read depth, referring to the number of reads that is found at a given genomic position. A relatively low average coverage of $0.07\times$ has been demonstrated as sufficient for accurate numerical chromosome analysis [30]. For monogenic disorders, sequencing at high coverage is required, which at this time is still too expensive for routine clinical applications at a whole-genome scale, and therefore various strategies aiming at affordable and rapid protocols are being developed. These protocols often provide a tandem solution combining genome-wide aneuploidy screening with PGT-M and can be classified in two groups, depending on whether sequencing data for the monogenic locus are derived with a targeted or a genome-wide method.

Targeted Sequencing

The two approaches presented here are merely an illustration of the wide range of possibilities (see also Chapter 6). A more affordable solution is to increase the read depth across the mutation site (minimum $100\times$) only. In one report, the mutation loci were captured in a preamplification reaction with mutation-specific primers while the concurrent inclusion of a specially designed primer pool allowed for parallel aneuploidy screening via real-time quantitative PCR [31]. The MARSALA method (mutated allele revealed by sequencing with aneuploidy and linkage analysis) works in a similar way: an aliquot of MALBAC-based WGA products undergoes targeted amplification and the mixture of WGA and targeted enriched templates is subsequently sequenced at low depth ($0.1–2\times$), yielding targeted SNP haplotyping results for PGT-M together with genome-wide PGT-A data [32]. In both examples, the targeted amplification is coupled with the need for a locus-specific preclinical workup.

Genome-Wide Sequencing

Genome-wide NGS is regarded as the most powerful platform for future PGT, as it will simultaneously offer genotype and chromosome copy number data with increased accuracy, reliability, and resolution, allowing a generic protocol for monogenic disorders (including the detection of *de novo* mutations and repeat expansions) and numerical and structural chromosomal aberrations (including balanced rearrangements). As the current cost is too high, the main approach has been to decrease the number of reads by reducing the complexity of the libraries. Some of these strategies are listed next (non-exhaustive).

The OnePGT solution, commercialized by Agilent, is an NGS-based generic application for PGT-M, PGT-SR, and PGT-A. The method takes advantage of reduced-representation genome sequencing in offering a single workflow, starting from MDA-based WGA and followed by library preparation with double restriction enzyme digestion and enrichment for fragments in a specific range of length; sequencing data interpretation relies on the haplarithmisis algorithm with concurrent chromosome copy number detection and SNP linkage-based haplotyping. The PGT-M module requires a minimum of 1.6× coverage and co-sequencing of samples from the parents and a valid reference family member.

Haploseek is another universal workflow offering an economical analysis of PGT-M and PGT-A within a 24-hour protocol, starting from PicoPLEX-based WGA and genome-wide low-coverage sequencing (0.3–1.4×) [33]. The information of high-quality whole-genome haplotypes of the couple and a reference obtained through SNP array is then integrated with the sample sequencing data, and a hidden Markov model is used to predict whether haplotypes of the samples are shared with the reference or not.

In another NGS approach, a target enrichment gene panel with nearly 5000 Mendelian disease-associated genes (TruSight One sequencing panel) was applied on MDA-based WGA products, thereby offering direct testing of family mutation(s) plus indirect mutation detection through haplotyping of SNPs together with chromosome copy number detection through the log ratio of signal intensities, i.e., PGT-M and PGT-A, all in a single workflow [34].

Further evaluation and thorough validation are required before any of these NGS-based approaches can be part of clinical PGT-M practice and wider application. In addition, it is clear that the implementation of comprehensive methods for PGT-M generates more complex genetic information which we currently do not fully understand; the innate embryo mosaicism, for instance, entails many ethical discussions and challenges for genetic counseling because we lack more knowledge to support data interpretation.

Competing Interests

The authors declare that they have no competing interests.

REFERENCES

1. Zegers-Hochschild F et al. The International Glossary on Infertility and Fertility Care, 2017. *Hum Reprod.* 2017;32:1786–801.
2. Handyside AH, Kontogianni EH, Hardy K, Winston RM. Pregnancies from biopsied human preimplantation embryos sexed by Y-specific DNA amplification. *Nature.* 1990;344:768–70.
3. Richards S et al. Standards and guidelines for the interpretation of sequence variants: A joint consensus recommendation of the American College of Medical Genetics and Genomics and the Association for Molecular Pathology. *Genet Med.* 2015;17:405–24.
4. Derks-Smeets IA et al. Hereditary breast and ovarian cancer and reproduction: An observational study on the suitability of preimplantation genetic diagnosis for both asymptomatic carriers and breast cancer survivors. *Breast Cancer Res Treat.* 2014;145:673–81.
5. Kuliev A et al. Preimplantation diagnosis and HLA typing for haemoglobin disorders. *Reprod Biomed Online.* 2005;11:362–70.
6. Kakourou G et al. The clinical utility of PGD with HLA matching: A collaborative multi-centre ESHRE study. *Hum Reprod.* 2018;33:520–30.
7. Van Rij MC et al. Preimplantation genetic diagnosis (PGD) for Huntington's disease: The experience of three European centres. *Eur J Hum Genet.* 2012;20:368–75.
8. Smeets HJ, Sallevelt SC, Dreesen JC, de Die-Smulders CE, de Coo IF. Preventing the transmission of mitochondrial DNA disorders using prenatal or preimplantation genetic diagnosis. *Ann N Y Acad Sci.* 2015;1350:29–36.
9. Zambelli F et al. Accurate and comprehensive analysis of single nucleotide variants and large deletions of the human mitochondrial genome in DNA and single cells. *Eur J Hum Genet.* 2017;25:1229–36.
10. Sallevelt SCEH et al. Preimplantation genetic diagnosis for mitochondrial DNA mutations: Analysis of one blastomere suffices. *J Med Genet.* 2017;54:693–7.

11. Heindryckx B et al. Mutation-free baby born from a mitochondrial encephalopathy, lactic acidosis and stroke-like syndrome carrier after blastocyst trophectoderm preimplantation genetic diagnosis. *Mitochondrion.* 2014;18:12–7.

12. Engelstad K et al. Attitudes toward prevention of mtDNA-related diseases through oocyte mitochondrial replacement therapy. *Hum Reprod.* 2016;31:1058–65.

13. Conboy I, Murthy N, Etienne J, Robinson Z. Making gene editing a therapeutic reality. *F1000Res.* 2018;7:pii: F1000 Faculty Rev-1970. doi: 10.12688/f1000research.16106.1. eCollection 2018.

14. Laurie AD et al. Preimplantation genetic diagnosis for hemophilia A using indirect linkage analysis and direct genotyping approaches. *J Thromb Haemost.* 2010;8:783–9.

15. Moutou C, Gardes N, Nicod JC, Viville S. Strategies and outcomes of PGD of familial adenomatous polyposis. *Mol Hum Reprod.* 2007;13:95–101.

16. Bermudez MG, Piyamongkol W, Tomaz S, Dudman E, Sherlock JK, Wells D. Single-cell sequencing and mini-sequencing for preimplantation genetic diagnosis. *Prenat Diagn.* 2003;23:669–77.

17. Traeger-Synodinos J et al. Blastocyst biopsy versus cleavage stage biopsy and blastocyst transfer for preimplantation genetic diagnosis of beta-thalassaemia: A pilot study. *Hum Reprod.* 2007;22:1443–49.

18. Renwick P, Trussler J, Lashwood A, Braude P, Ogilvie CM. Preimplantation genetic haplotyping: 127 diagnostic cycles demonstrating a robust, efficient alternative to direct mutation testing on single cells. *Reprod Biomed Online.* 2010;20:470–6.

19. Coskun S, Alsmadi O. Whole genome amplification from a single cell: A new era for preimplantation genetic diagnosis. *Prenat Diagn.* 2007;27:297–302.

20. Spits C et al. Whole-genome multiple displacement amplification from single cells. *Nat Protoc.* 2006;1:1965–70.

21. Langmore JP. Rubicon Genomics, Inc. *Pharmacogenomics.* 2002;3:557–60.

22. Zong C, Lu S, Chapman AR, Xie XS. Genome-wide detection of single-nucleotide and copy-number variations of a single human cell. *Science.* 2012;338:1622–6.

23. Deleye L et al. Whole genome amplification with SurePlex results in better copy number alteration detection using sequencing data compared to the MALBAC method. *Sci Rep.* 2015;5:11711.

24. de Bourcy CF, De Vlaminck I, Kanbar JN, Wang J, Gawad C, Quake SR. A quantitative comparison of single-cell whole genome amplification methods. *PLOS ONE.* 2014;9:e105585.

25. Deleye L, Gansemans Y, De Coninck D, Van Nieuwerburgh F, Deforce D. Massively parallel sequencing of micro-manipulated cells targeting a comprehensive panel of disease-causing genes: A comparative evaluation of upstream whole-genome amplification methods. *PLOS ONE.* 2018;13(4):e0196334.

26. LaFramboise T. Single nucleotide polymorphism arrays: A decade of biological, computational and technological advances. *Nucleic Acids Res.* 2009;37:4181–93.

27. Handyside AH et al. Karyomapping: A universal method for genome wide analysis of genetic disease based on mapping crossovers between parental haplotypes. *J Med Genet.* 2010;47:651–8.

28. Natesan SA et al. Genome-wide karyomapping accurately identifies the inheritance of single-gene defects in human preimplantation embryos *in vitro. Genet Med.* 2014;16:838–45.

29. Zamani Esteki M et al. Concurrent whole-genome haplotyping and copy-number profiling of single cells. *Am J Hum Genet.* 2015;96:894–912.

30. Yin X et al. Massively parallel sequencing for chromosomal abnormality testing in trophectoderm cells of human blastocysts. *Biol Reprod.* 2013;88:69.

31. Treff NR, Fedick A, Tao X, Devkota B, Taylor D, Scott RT Jr. Evaluation of targeted next-generation sequencing-based preimplantation genetic diagnosis of monogenic disease. *Fertil Steril.* 2013;99:1377–84.

32. Yan L et al. Live births after simultaneous avoidance of monogenic diseases and chromosome abnormality by next-generation sequencing with linkage analyses. *Proc Natl Acad Sci U S A.* 2015;112:15964–9.

33. Backenroth D et al. Haploseek: A 24-hour all-in-one method for preimplantation genetic diagnosis (PGD) of monogenic disease and aneuploidy. *Genet Med.* 2019;21:1390–9.

34. Del Rey J et al. Novel double factor PGT strategy analyzing blastocyst stage embryos in a single NGS procedure. *PLOS ONE.* 2018;13(10):e0205692.

6

Novel Methods in Preimplantation Genetic Testing: Comprehensive Preimplantation Genetic Testing

Olga Tsuiko and Joris Robert Vermeesch

CONTENTS

Comprehensive PGT: Introduction

Since the first application in the 1990s [1], PGT-M is now performed worldwide to avoid the transmission of Mendelian hereditary conditions that run in the family to the offspring. At the same time, the development of microarray-based technologies and later implementation of next-generation sequencing (NGS), which allow genome-wide chromosome screening for aneuploidy, has facilitated the use of PGT-A to select against embryos with unbalanced karyotype. Traditionally, patients have been referred either to PGT-M/PGT-SR or PGT-A, based on medical indication, but no combined tests have been performed. However, couples undergoing PGT-M can have "unaffected" embryos for a single-gene disorder, but because of high aneuploidy rate in human IVF embryos [2], the seemingly healthy embryos can carry chromosomal aberrations that can lead to implantation failure or adverse pregnancy outcome. For this reason, couples can benefit from PGT-M in conjunction with PGT-A (further referred to as comprehensive PGT), selecting only those embryos that are free of disease and have a normal euploid karyotype. In the past decade, different strategies have been implemented to allow simultaneous detection of monogenic and chromosomal disorders. One of the first attempts to do so used the two-biopsy approach: (i) oocyte polar body was biopsied for chromosome screening via array comparative genomic hybridization (aCGH) and (ii) day 3 biopsy was performed for genetic analysis for cystis fibrosis or von Hippel-Lindau disease using multiplex PCR [3,4]. Later, the use of whole-genome amplified (WGA) product for comprehensive embryo testing made it possible to perform SNP microarray analysis for aneuploidy and PCR-based linkage analysis for GM1 gangliosidoses from the same biopsied material [5]. By combining the data from two independent assays, five embryos out of ten were suitable for transfer, as they were both euploid and disease-free. This approach was later extended to a variety of genetic disorders, and the first systematic analysis demonstrated improved pregnancy rates from 45.4% to 68.4% and a reduction in spontaneous abortion rate from 15.5% to 5.5%, which was especially evident in patients with advanced maternal age [6]. The same beneficial effect of comprehensive PGT was also observed in a recent large-scale study, demonstrating the increase of clinical pregnancy rate per transfer from 33.6% to 49% by avoiding transferring of embryos with low developmental potential [7].

Genome-Wide Haplotyping for Comprehensive PGT

Despite successful implementation of different technologies for PGT-M coupled with PGT-A, previous studies have relied mostly on two separate protocols for sample processing. Moreover, traditional targeted PCR-based assays for PGT-M are time- and labor-intensive and require an extensive workup, which can lead to elevated costs and long waiting lists. In addition, PCR assays need to minimize allele dropout (ADO) effect, which is one of the main causes of misdiagnosis. The recent advent of high-throughput single-cell genotyping technologies has revolutionized preimplantation genetic testing by overcoming the limitations of conventional methods. Simultaneous interrogation of hundreds of thousands of informative single-nucleotide polymorphisms (SNPs) across the entire genome of an embryo has shifted the clinical practice from the traditional single-locus methods to the use of genome-wide haplotyping of single cells that make it possible to (i) determine the inheritance of parental disease-associated alleles in the embryo and (ii) perform copy-number profiling [8]. To date, two genome-wide haplotyping methods have been developed that use SNP array data: karyomapping [9] and haplarithmisis, which is integrated into single-cell haplotyping and imputation of linked disease variants (siCHILD) computational workflow [10]. Both methodologies use the linkage disequilibrium principle to infer disease-causing mutations and assign them to parental haplotype blocks across all chromosomes (Figure 6.1), thus they involve genotyping and genome-wide SNP analysis of parental DNA, whole-genome amplified embryo DNA, and DNA

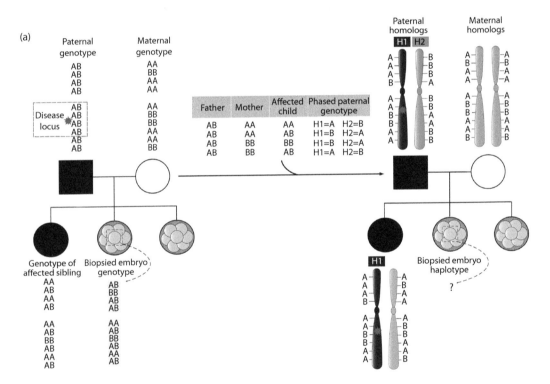

FIGURE 6.1 Principles of genome-wide haplotyping for comprehensive PGT. Clinically implemented embryo haplotyping methods for PGT-M are used to deduce the inheritance of disease-associated parental alleles by the embryo, using discrete SNP genotypes (AA, BB, or AB) derived from the parents and phasing reference. (a) An example of a family with an autosomal dominant disorder where both the father and the child carry a disease locus. First, DNA from parents, a child (phasing reference), and WGA embryo biopsy are genotyped using SNP arrays. Next, informative SNPs are retrieved from the parents, which are characterized as heterozygous in one parent and homozygous in the other. The use of informative SNPs and affected child's genotype makes it possible to phase parental genotypes and determine the transmission of paternal and maternal homologs. For simplicity, only paternal-informative SNPs are depicted in this case, and based on phased paternal genotype, the child inherited paternal homolog 1 (H1) with a causative mutation, while paternal H2 carries a normal allele.   *(Continued)*

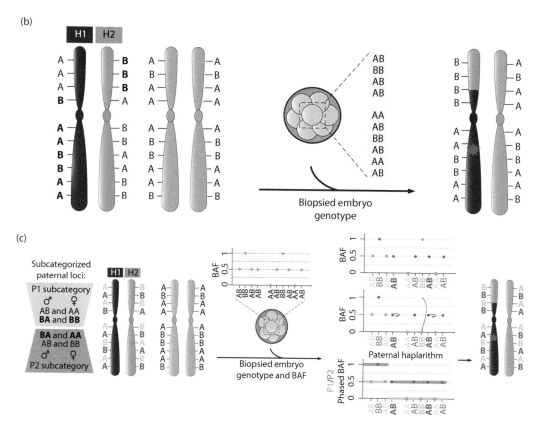

FIGURE 6.1 (CONTINUED) Principles of genome-wide haplotyping for comprehensive PGT. (b) Subsequently, parental haplotype information is used to infer the inheritance of mutant or normal alleles in the embryo, using discrete genotypes of biopsied cells. Genotypes, depicted in bold in the father, indicate transmitted paternal homologs in the embryo, which in this case inherited the disease-associated H1 and is not suitable for transfer. This approach is used by karyomapping [9], which also makes it possible to identify homologous recombination sites. In addition, adjusted phasing rules make it possible to eliminate random WGA artifacts that can result in Mendelian inconsistencies. (c) Alternatively, haplarithmisis [10] uses SNP B-allele frequency (BAF) values instead of discrete SNP genotypes for single-cell haplotyping. Based on the defined phased parental genotype combinations, the SNP–BAF values of an embryo are binned into paternal-informative SNP subcategories P1 (blue box) and P2 (red box); a similar approach is used for maternal-informative SNPs to obtain maternal M1 and M2 subcategories (not shown). When the cell inherits H1 from the father, and either H1 or H2 from the mother, the P1 SNP–BAFs have values of either 0 or 1 (corresponding to homozygous AA and BB genotypes in the cell, respectively) and the P2 SNP–BAFs have a value of 0.5 (corresponding to heterozygous AB genotypes in the cell). In contrast, when the cell inherits H2 from the father, the P1 SNP–BAFs have a value of 0.5 and the P2 SNP–BAFs have a value of either 0 or 1. A defined subset of the single-cell BAF values (paternal BA genotypes, indicated in bold) are then mirrored around the 0.5 axis (indicated with arrows), making it possible to segment single-cell P1 and P2 BAF values for consecutive SNPs in the genome. The resulting P1 and P2 BAF segments (depicted in blue and red, respectively) now define the haplotype blocks inherited from paternal H1 and H2. For H1 loci, P1 and P2 SNP–BAF segments have values of 0 and 0.5, respectively, and for H2 loci P1 and P2 have values of 0.5 and 1, respectively. The reconstructed haplotype blocks of the cell can be used to determine the transmission of mutant or normal allele in the embryo. Because this approach uses single-cell BAF values, concomitant embryo copy number profiling is also performed.

derived from a close relative, e.g., child or both parents of the affected couple. Although the downstream computational workflow bears some differences, parental genotypes first need to be phased via SNP genotype calls derived from a close relative in both approaches, after which paternal and maternal homologs are established. First, informative SNPs are identified, which are defined as heterozygous in one parent and homozygous in the other. These informative loci are arranged into strings of consecutive SNPs on each homolog with the use of a reference genotype from a close relative, thus establishing a "phase" (Figure 6.1a). Following genome-wide phasing, the disease-associated alleles are then linked to a parental haplotype, which can subsequently be traced back in the embryo (Figure 6.1b, c).

Genome-wide haplotyping approaches used in karyomapping and haplarithmisis have several advantages over conventional methods. First, both methods are generic and can diagnose any familial transmitted Mendelian disorder with a known cause, thus precluding the need for development and optimization of targeted locus- or family-specific protocols. Because the analysis is performed on a genome-wide scale, simultaneous screening for multiple Mendelian disorders and traits is possible. Second, both methods minimize the issues associated with random ADO and allele drop-in (ADI) because of WGA artifacts, which is a common problem of PCR-based targeted assays. The inheritance of DNA mutations is deducted from the reconstructed haplotypes in the embryo, so there is no direct mutation analysis. For this reason, even if some polymorphic markers will result in ADO, the significant part of variants, flanking the locus of interest, will remain. Third, meiotic homologous recombination sites can be accurately identified, which can break down the linkage of pathogenic variant with its nearby SNPs. Finally, the ability to also detect genome-wide copy-number aberrations makes it possible to perform comprehensive PGT for monogenic disorders, chromosomal structural rearrangements, and aneuploidy screening in a single assay. Importantly, the use of SNP array data combined with sophisticated computational workflow enables identification of uniparental disomies (UPDs), which can either lead to imprinting-related disorders, such as Angelman/Prader-Willi syndromes, or loss of heterozygosity can unmask a disease-causing recessive mutation. In addition, in the case of balanced translocation carriers, both methods can also distinguish between embryos with chromosomally normal genome and embryos that are carriers of balanced rearrangements.

Due to the described attractive features that address the issues of FISH- and PCR-based assays, karyomapping and haplarithmisis have been successfully implemented into the clinical practice for embryo selection [11–13]. The main difference between the two genome-wide approaches is that karyomapping only uses discrete SNP calls, thus it struggles with the reliable detection of post-zygotic mitotic chromosome gains. It has been well established that cleavage-stage IVF embryos are prone to mitotic chromosome mis-segregations [2,14–17], which can contribute to chromosomal mosaicism, observed at the blastocyst stage [18–24]. Therefore, the inability to detect mitotic trisomies can prohibit the use of karyomapping for comprehensive chromosome screening. In contrast, haplarithmisis overcomes this limitation, as it also uses continuous B-allele frequency (BAF) values, which consequently make it possible to distinguish meiotic errors from mitotic ones and reveal the parental origin of aneuploidy [10]. In turn, this can bring additional benefits for embryo ranking: in the case of meiotic errors, all the cells of an embryo will contain oocyte- or sperm-derived aneuploidy, and such an embryo will not be chosen for transfer; in the case of mitotic aneuploidy, only a subset of cells will be affected, but they can contribute to implantation failure or first-trimester miscarriage [20,23], and such an embryo will have a lower ranking priority. In addition, by using haplarithmisis, we have unraveled a wide range of genomic anomalies such as mixoploidy/chimerism in the embryo, including dispermic fertilization, polar body fusion, and segregation of blastomeres to androgenetic and gynogenetic cell lineages upon post-zygotic cellular divisions [25,26]. Hence understanding the origin and the extent of aneuploidy can leverage embryo prioritization and selection for transfer [12,27]. Recently, we have also shown that 0PN and 1PN zygotes, which are normally discarded from further clinical use, can develop into balanced diploid embryos [28]. This observation challenges the current embryo selection guidelines against the use of 0PN and 1PN zygotes, as the inclusion of such zygotes for comprehensive PGT can increase the number of available embryos for transfer per single IVF-PGT cycle by over 20%.

Alternative Phasing Approaches

Despite the clinical value of genome-wide haplotyping-based approaches, in a minority of cases the references required to phase the parental genomes are unavailable, and comprehensive PGT cannot be applied in these families. These cases often involve either couples with a dominant disorder whose parents are deceased, or couples with *de novo* mutations who do not have children yet. As an alternative, it has been proposed that other affected relatives could be used for phasing. Because full siblings share on average 50% of their genome [29], 50% of the embryonic haplotype structure can be inferred by using parental siblings as a phasing reference. We have recently developed an alternative phasing approach using parental siblings (e.g., brother or sister) for comprehensive PGT by implementing the identity-by-state (IBS) principle, which measures the sharing of alleles between individuals based on the genotype data [40]. By comparing SNP genotype data, IBS can be assigned to three possible categories: (i) the genotypes between two individuals are completely identical (AA/AA, BB/BB, or AB/AB) and are assigned to IBS2 (=2 shared alleles); (ii) the compared genotypes share one allele (AA/AB, BB/AB, AB/AA, or AB/BB) and are assigned to IBS1 (=1 shared allele), and (iii) the compared genotypes are completely distinct (AA/BB or BB/AA) and are assigned to IBS0 (=0 alleles shared) (Figure 6.2). By embedding the modified pipeline into the haplarithmisis workflow, genome-wide haplotyping for PGT-M was possible for loci of shared heterozygous IBS1 regions and the method achieved a 100% diagnostic concordance rate, compared to the standard parent-offspring trio phasing [40]. Importantly, the IBS-based analytical concept overcomes a significant limitation of the identity-by-descent (IBD)-based "common allele" tracing approach, where only relatives carrying the disease-causing allele can be used. In contrast, in the IBS-based approach both affected and unaffected parental siblings can be used for haplotype block reconstruction in embryos. Consequently, this novel strategy for PGT-M can be beneficial for those families who do not have an available reference material and who would otherwise not be able to seek genome-wide linkage analysis–based PGT-M. In some social or cultural contexts, the use of parental siblings can also ease the discomfort of disclosing the reproductive history of the couple to their parents.

Haplotyping-by-Sequencing for Comprehensive PGT

Until now, both karyomapping and haplarithmisis relied on SNP array data, but the rapid uptake of massive parallel sequencing has paved the way to new diagnostic opportunities in reproductive medicine. Low-coverage sequencing has been well implemented in routine clinical practice for PGT-A, and targeted NGS-based protocols have also been developed for PGT-M [30,31]. Novel NGS-based protocols have also been developed for comprehensive PGT to detect both aneuploidy and single-gene disorders. One such approach, mutated allele revealed by sequencing with aneuploidy and linkage analysis (MARSALA), combines low-coverage genome sequencing for aneuploidy with low-coverage targeted sequencing for haplotype phasing [32]. This method has been successfully applied in the clinic to select against single-base mutation on the autosome and the X-chromosome [32,33]. Similar to conventional targeted protocols, the main disadvantage of targeted haplotyping is the need for custom targeted sequencing assays. To overcome this, a novel universal NGS-based workflow was introduced, called Haploseek, which provides haplotype and copy-number information in single cells using a custom hidden Markov model [34]. Haploseek pipeline has been retrospectively applied to analyze blastomere and/or blastocyst biopsies for PGT-SR, demonstrating concordant results with a conventional two-step diagnostic approach. In addition, we have recently developed an alternative and cost-effective genome-wide single-cell haplotyping approach, using the genotyping-by-sequencing (GBS) methodology [35]. The GBS protocol combines restriction-enzyme-mediated genome complexity and size reduction, GBS library construction, and multiplex NGS for high-density SNP discovery and mapping. The obtained GBS sequencing data is then converted to the SNP array type data, i.e., genotypes, BAF- and logR-values, and applied to the haplarithmisis workflow to allow genome-wide linkage analysis via suitable phasing references. Today, both SNP array and GBS-based computational pipelines of haplarithmisis have also been integrated into the interactive web platform, termed haplarithm inference of variant alleles (HiVA) [35]. Moreover, an adaptation of the GBS-based workflow has been commercialized as OnePGT (Agilent Technologies), and the method has been fully verified and validated in a retrospective multicenter study [41].

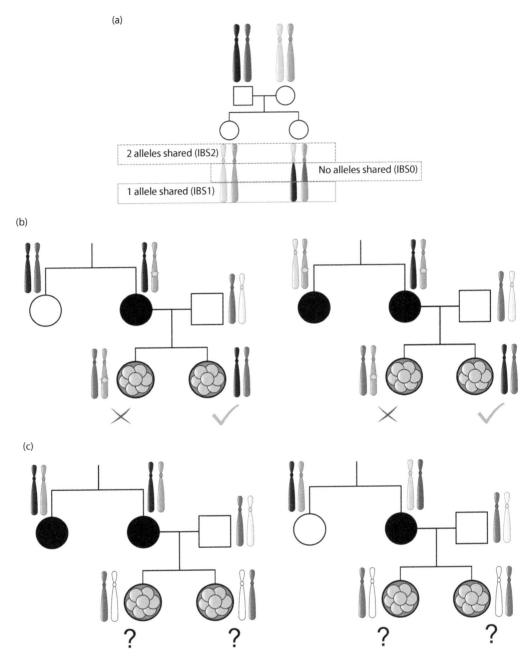

FIGURE 6.2 Alternative phasing for comprehensive PGT. Embryo haplotyping for comprehensive PGT can also be performed using parental siblings by applying the principle of identity-by-state (IBS). (a) The IBS regions are first identified between the two sibling pairs and categorized into IBS0 (no alleles shared), IBS1 (one shared allele), and IBS2 (both alleles shared). Subsequently, phasing and transmission of alleles in the embryo can be performed based on informative IBS1 regions. (b) An example of a family where an affected mother has disease-associated allele, while her sister is healthy (left). Because the affected mother and the healthy sister share one allele, it is possible to deduce which of the alleles is normal and which one is mutated, hence embryo haplotyping can be performed using IBS1 regions. If biopsied embryo cells will contain the disease-associated allele from the mother (pink), the embryo will be classified as affected. The same approach can be performed when both the mother and the sister carry the disease-associated locus (right). (c) If the mutation lies in the non-informative IBS2 (left) or IBS0 (right) regions, the disease locus cannot be identified and embryo haplotyping cannot be performed.

Future Directions

The newly developed haplotyping-by-sequencing technologies require family members for phasing and are currently not suitable for the detection of *de novo* mutations that occurred in the prospective parents. To overcome these issues, generic strategies for genome-wide haplotyping are currently being pioneered. For example, the long fragment read (LFR) technology can generate the long-range phased variants, achieved through the stochastic separation of long parental DNA fragments into physically distinct pools. Each pool contains a fraction of the haploid genome, which is then whole-genome amplified, fragmented, and converted to a unique barcode short-read sequencing library. Following pooling and sequencing of the barcoded DNA libraries derived from the same sample, genetic variants can be assigned to parental haplotypes [36]. Using LFR technology, blastocyst biopsies have been analyzed and 82% of all *de novo* changes have been detected in human IVF embryos [37]. Another approach uses a microfluidic device capable of separating and amplifying homolog chromosomes of single-metaphase cells, making it possible to retrieve haplotypes of each individual chromosome [38]. Finally, microfluidics-based linked-read sequencing technology may also open new horizons for direct genome phasing and haplotyping. The technology relies on a droplet generation system that molecularly barcodes long genomic DNA and prepares libraries, using microfluidics. The generated libraries are compatible with standard short-read sequencing. Because each droplet contains an individual DNA molecule with unique barcoded primers, short DNA fragments containing the same barcode can then be computationally linked back to each other, reconstructing long-range haplotypes [39]. Although the current high costs of these proof-of-concept methods can prohibit them from routine clinical practice, we envision a profound impact of long- and linked-read sequencing technologies on future PGT to enable direct phasing and eliminate the need for analyzing additional family members.

REFERENCES

1. Handyside AH, Kontogianni EH, Hardy K, Winston RML. Pregnancies from biopsied human preimplantation embryos sexed by Y-specific DNA amplification. *Nature.* 19 Apr, 1990;344(6268):768–70.
2. Vanneste E et al. Chromosome instability is common in human cleavage-stage embryos. *Nat Med.* 26 May, 2009;15(5):577–83.
3. Obradors A et al. Birth of a healthy boy after a double factor PGD in a couple carrying a genetic disease and at risk for aneuploidy: Case Report. *Hum Reprod.* 15 May, 2008;23(8):1949–56.
4. Obradors A et al. Outcome of twin babies free of Von Hippel-Lindau disease after a double-factor preimplantation genetic diagnosis: Monogenetic mutation analysis and comprehensive aneuploidy screening. *Fertil Steril.* Mar 2009;91(3):933.e1–e7.
5. Brezina PR et al. Single-gene testing combined with single nucleotide polymorphism microarray preimplantation genetic diagnosis for aneuploidy: A novel approach in optimizing pregnancy outcome. *Fertil Steril.* 1 Apr, 2011;95(5):1786.e5–.e8.
6. Rechitsky S, Pakhalchuk T, San Ramos G, Goodman A, Zlatopolsky Z, Kuliev A. First systematic experience of preimplantation genetic diagnosis for single-gene disorders, and/or preimplantation human leukocyte antigen typing, combined with 24-chromosome aneuploidy testing. *Fertil Steril.* Feb 2015;103(2):503–12.
7. Minasi MG et al. Genetic diseases and aneuploidies can be detected with a single blastocyst biopsy: A successful clinical approach. *Hum Reprod.* 1 Aug, 2017;32(8):1770–7.
8. Vermeesch JR, Voet T, Devriendt K. Prenatal and pre-implantation genetic diagnosis. *Nat Rev Genet.* Oct 1, 2016;17(10):643–56.
9. Handyside AH et al. Karyomapping: A universal method for genome wide analysis of genetic disease based on mapping crossovers between parental haplotypes. *J Med Genet.* 1 Oct, 2010;47(10):651–8.
10. Zamani Esteki M et al. Concurrent whole-genome haplotyping and copy-number profiling of single cells. *Am J Hum Genet.* 4 Jun, 2015;96(6):894–912.
11. Ben-Nagi J et al. Karyomapping: A single centre's experience from application of methodology to ongoing pregnancy and live-birth rates. *Reprod Biomed Online.* Sep 2017;35(3):264–71.

12. Dimitriadou E et al. Principles guiding embryo selection following genome-wide haplotyping of preimplantation embryos. *Hum Reprod.* 1 Mar, 2017;32(3):687–97.

13. Konstantinidis M et al. Live births following Karyomapping of human blastocysts: Experience from clinical application of the method. *Reprod Biomed Online.* Sep 2015;31(3):394–403.

14. Johnson DS et al. Preclinical validation of a microarray method for full molecular karyotyping of blastomeres in a 24-h protocol. *Hum Reprod.* Apr 2010;25(4):1066–75.

15. Chavez SL et al. Dynamic blastomere behaviour reflects human embryo ploidy by the four-cell stage. *Nat Commun.* 4 Jan, 2012;3(1):1251.

16. Chow JF, Yeung WS, Lau EY, Lee VC, Ng EH, Ho P-C. Array comparative genomic hybridization analyses of all blastomeres of a cohort of embryos from young IVF patients revealed significant contribution of mitotic errors to embryo mosaicism at the cleavage stage. *Reprod Biol Endocrinol.* 24 Nov, 2014;12(1):105.

17. Mertzanidou A et al. Microarray analysis reveals abnormal chromosomal complements in over 70% of 14 normally developing human embryos. *Hum Reprod.* 1 Jan, 2013;28(1):256–64.

18. Vera-Rodríguez M et al. Distribution patterns of segmental aneuploidies in human blastocysts identified by next-generation sequencing. *Fertil Steril.* Apr 2016;105(4):1047–55.e2.

19. Capalbo A, Rienzi L. Mosaicism between trophectoderm and inner cell mass. *Fertil Steril.* May 2017;107(5):1098–106.

20. Fragouli E et al. Analysis of implantation and ongoing pregnancy rates following the transfer of mosaic diploid–aneuploid blastocysts. *Hum Genet.* 9 Jul, 2017;136(7):805–19.

21. Ruttanajit T et al. Detection and quantitation of chromosomal mosaicism in human blastocysts using copy number variation sequencing. *Prenat Diagn.* 1 Feb, 2016;36(2):154–62.

22. Munné S, Wells D. Detection of mosaicism at blastocyst stage with the use of high-resolution next-generation sequencing. *Fertil Steril.* 1 May, 2017;107(5):1085–91.

23. Munné S et al. Detailed investigation into the cytogenetic constitution and pregnancy outcome of replacing mosaic blastocysts detected with the use of high-resolution next-generation sequencing. *Fertil Steril.* 1 Jul, 2017;108(1):62–71.e8.

24. Spinella F et al. Extent of chromosomal mosaicism influences the clinical outcome of *in vitro* fertilization treatments. *Fertil Steril.* Jan 2018;109(1):77–83.

25. Tšuiko O et al. Genome stability of bovine *in vivo*-conceived cleavage-stage embryos is higher compared to *in vitro*-produced embryos. *Hum Reprod.* 1 Nov, 2017;32(11):2348–57.

26. Destouni A et al. Zygotes segregate entire parental genomes in distinct blastomere lineages causing cleavage-stage chimerism and mixoploidy. *Genome Res.* 2016;26(5):567–78.

27. Grati FR, Gallazzi G, Branca L, Maggi F, Simoni G, Yaron Y. An evidence-based scoring system for prioritizing mosaic aneuploid embryos following preimplantation genetic screening. *Reprod Biomed Online.* Apr 2018;36(4):442–9.

28. Destouni A et al. Genome-wide haplotyping embryos developing from 0PN and 1PN zygotes increases transferrable embryos in PGT-M. *Hum Reprod.* 1 Dec, 2018;33(12):2302–11.

29. Gagnon A, Beise J, Vaupel JW. Genome-wide identity-by-descent sharing among CEPH siblings. *Genet Epidemiol.* 1 Nov, 2005;29(3):215–24.

30. Treff NR, Fedick A, Tao X, Devkota B, Taylor D, Scott RT. Evaluation of targeted next-generation sequencing–based preimplantation genetic diagnosis of monogenic disease. *Fertil Steril.* Apr 2013;99(5):1377–84.e6.

31. Kubikova N, Babariya D, Sarasa J, Spath K, Alfarawati S, Wells D. Clinical application of a protocol based on universal next-generation sequencing for the diagnosis of beta-thalassaemia and sickle cell anaemia in preimplantation embryos. *Reprod Biomed Online.* 1 Aug, 2018;37(2):136–44.

32. Yan L et al. Live births after simultaneous avoidance of monogenic diseases and chromosome abnormality by next-generation sequencing with linkage analyses. *Proc Natl Acad Sci U S A.* 29 Dec, 2015;112(52):15964–9.

33. Ren Y et al. Clinical applications of MARSALA for preimplantation genetic diagnosis of spinal muscular atrophy. *J Genet Genomics.* 20 Sep, 2016;43(9):541–7.

34. Backenroth D et al. Haploseek: A 24-hour all-in-one method for preimplantation genetic diagnosis (PGD) of monogenic disease and aneuploidy. *Genet Med.* 19 Nov, 2018;1.

35. Esteki MZ et al. HiVA: An integrative wet- and dry-lab platform for haplotype and copy number analysis of single-cell genomes. *bioRxiv.* 7 Mar, 2019;564914.

36. Peters BA et al. Accurate whole-genome sequencing and haplotyping from 10 to 20 human cells. *Nature.* 12 Jul, 2012;487(7406):190–5.
37. Peters BA et al. Detection and phasing of single base *de novo* mutations in biopsies from human *in vitro* fertilized embryos by advanced whole-genome sequencing. *Genome Res.* 11 Mar, 2015;25(3):426–34.
38. Fan HC, Wang J, Potanina A, Quake SR. Whole-genome molecular haplotyping of single cells. *Nat Biotechnol.* 19 Jan, 2011;29(1):51–7.
39. Zheng GXY et al. Haplotyping germline and cancer genomes with high-throughput linked-read sequencing. *Nat Biotechnol.* 1 Mar, 2016;34(3):303–11.
40. Ding J et al. Identity-by-state based haplotyping expands the application of comprehensive preimplantation genetic testing. *Hum Reprod.* Mar 27, 2020;35(3):718–26.
41. Masset H et al. Multi-centre evaluation of a comprehensive preimplantation genetic test through haplotyping-by-sequencing. *Hum Reprod.* Aug 1, 2019;34(8):1608–19.

7

Time-Lapse Imaging and Preimplantation Genetic Testing

Alison Campbell

CONTENTS

Microscopic Observation of the *in Vitro* Human Embryo

During fertility treatment, morphological assessment of the preimplantation human embryo is the most established and simple approach to guide embryo selection. The correlation between embryo morphology and implantation potential has been extensively demonstrated and documented, but this series of swift microscopic manual assessments of morphology is increasingly being considered a relatively poor indicator of an embryo's potential to result in a healthy live birth, even if selection takes place at the blastocyst stage [1].

Morphological embryo assessment typically consists of several sequential, timed daily microscopic observations, and ranking of them is commonly guided by professional body or consensus guidelines. Using such systems, the preimplantation cleavage stage embryo is assessed primarily on cell number and degree of cytoplasmic fragmentation, as well as developmental stage, with a demonstrated association with viability [2–4]. These embryo observations, however, employed to limit exposure to and potential stress caused by the assessment environment, provide limited information on developmental rates or patterns and little insight into the chromosomal complement of the embryo.

This established morphological approach to human preimplantation embryo assessment and selection has evolved in recent years with the introduction of time-lapse monitoring, enabling the kinetics and transient behaviors of embryo development to also be assessed, with reports of improved embryo selection and clinical outcomes using this "morphokinetic" information [5].

Time-Lapse Imaging of the Human Embryo *in Vitro*

Several time-lapse incubation devices are now commercially available for the IVF laboratory. They are designed to capture images of the fertilizing and developing embryos at regular intervals (commonly 5–20 minutes apart) throughout the *in-vitro* culture period, avoiding the need to remove the embryos from the protected and optimized environment for visual microscopic assessment. The Embryoscope™ (Vitrolife, Sweden) was the first instrument to provide this relatively stable, "uninterrupted" incubation combined with internal microscopy as an alternative to a standard IVF incubator. The introduction of such time-lapse devices has resulted in a plethora of reports describing human preimplantation embryo development in greater detail, with descriptions of both its theoretical and demonstrable impact on embryo selection and clinical outcomes [6–8].

Time-lapse monitoring of the dynamics of embryo development, often in association with conventional qualitative morphological observations, provides detailed morphokinetic information on individual embryos. These data, consisting of timings, morphologies, irregularities, and durations of embryo developmental events, can be retrospectively analyzed against outcome measures, such as blastulation, implantation, embryo ploidy, or healthy live birth. These data can also be used to derive predictive selection models, or algorithms, or simple preferential selection (or deselection) criteria, for prospective use in the IVF laboratory. Meseguer et al., in 2012, first reported a 20% increase in pregnancy rate using time-lapse systems compared with standard incubation, and attributed this improvement to the stable culture conditions of the time-lapse device, and use of morphokinetic variables for embryo selection [5]. More recently, several large studies and randomized controlled trials have also reported improvements when time-lapse algorithms were used for embryo selection, compared with morphology alone [9].

Time-Lapse Data Collection and Handling

Although automated, or semi-automated, time-lapse video analysis and interpretation is likely to be increasingly used in the future, data generated from these devices has so far primarily come from manual image assessment and recordings of the events observed (i.e., by "annotation"), on human review of the time-lapse images viewed as videos. Due to the manual nature of data collection, to minimize subjectivity and maximize data quality, rigorous training of practitioners and quality assurance is required to assure the output and value of a clinical time-lapse offering [10]. The use of intracorrelation coefficients enables assessment of different practitioners and reproducibility of annotations of the morphokinetic variables. Sundvall and colleagues considered inter- and intrapractitioner variation in annotation using this intra-class correlation coefficient, and demonstrated close correlation between experienced and newer time-lapse users for most morphokinetic variables, but highlighted that some "static morphologic parameters," such as multinucleation and blastomere evenness, were at risk of subjectivity [11].

Where there are multiple practitioners involved in time-lapse data collection, the risk of subjectivity and inconsistency are enhanced, and intrapractitioner annotation variation may also exist. Minimization of this subjectivity can be achieved by clear definition of key variables and with strict annotation practice set out within the standard operating procedure (SOP). Guidelines for nomenclature and annotation are available to encourage international consistency and to allow compilation of large data in the future [12].

The most commonly recorded morphokinetic variables follow the basic principles of human embryology and mitosis, and include timing of pronuclear appearance and fading, increasing cell numbers (time to 2, 3, 4, 5, 6 cells, etc.), assessment of fragmentation, cell evenness, synchronicity and nucleation, and the times to reach—and durations of—embryo differentiation to the morula and blastocyst stages (Figure 7.1).

Selection for intrauterine transfer of the most viable embryo from a cohort in assisted reproduction technology (ART) is essential to minimize the time taken to reach pregnancy and successful delivery of a healthy child. With increasing female age being the most negatively impactful variable associated with fertility, failure to choose the best embryo the first time could not only prolong the patient pathway and introduce emotional and financial burden, but could also reduce the chances of successful outcomes during future attempts at IVF by delaying this process, as maternal age advances.

Time-lapse (morphokinetic) analysis alone is considered by many to provide superior embryo selection to traditional and static morphology, and time-lapse selection algorithms have been developed, published, and independently evaluated, although reports of their performance, compared with traditional morphological selection, and their transferability between clinical settings, is inconsistent, in part due to lack of standardization and the heterogeneity in its application [13]. Recently, deep learning has been implemented in several areas of medicine. It has also been proposed as a superior automated and

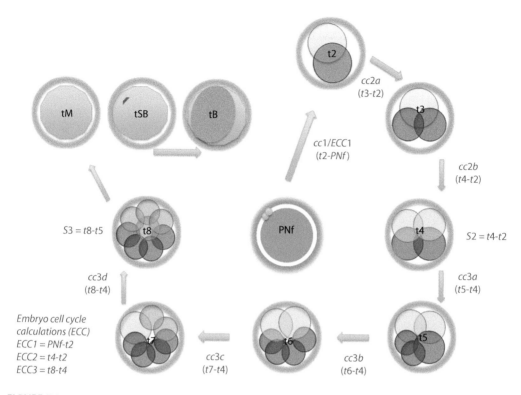

FIGURE 7.1 Schematic of standard morphokinetic variables. Times (t) from insemination to pronuclear fading (PNf) through each cell division to eight cells (t2 to t8), morula (tM), start of blastulation (tSB), and the full blastocyst stage (tB). Rounds of cell division are coded as embryo cell cycles (ECC); when cell number doubles (e.g., from four to eight) and the blastomere cell cycles are coded as "cc"; the numbers represent sequential divisions and the letters represent the individual blastomeres. (From Campbell A. Chapter 3 in *Atlas of Time Lapse Embryology*. Boca Raton, FL; CRC Press; 2015. With permission.)

standardized approach to facilitate embryo selection, using photographic data from time-lapse imaging. A large multicenter retrospective analysis of over 10,000 embryos used a deep learning trained model to predict clinical pregnancy with an average area under the curve (AUC) of the receiver operating characteristic (ROC) curve of 0.93 (95% CI 0.92–0.94). Prospective studies are required in order to assess the potential clinical impact of this approach, which promises to offer an automated method to improve identification of the embryo(s) from a cohort with the highest propensity for implantation [14].

Selection and Deselection Morphokinetic Criteria

In addition to enabling detailed, time-stamped monitoring of the morphokinetics of embryo development, time-lapse technology also allows the identification of aberrant embryo cleavage events, which may not be observable using "snapshot" traditional static microscopy methods. Potentially the most valuable example of aberrant cleavage, and one of the most well reported in terms of its correlation with viability, is the phenomenon of a multiple, as opposed to dichotomous, cleavage of a blastomere to three or more daughter cells. Several studies have demonstrated the ability of time-lapse to identify such aberrant cleavage divisions and highlight the reduced implantation potential of these embryos, compared with their counterparts that mitotically divide into two daughter cells. In a cohort of 1659 transferred embryos, the incidence of this "direct division" (occurring within 5 hours) was 13.7%, and the implantation rate of these embryos was markedly and statistically significantly lower than for embryos with a normal cleavage pattern (1.2% vs. 20.2%, respectively) [6]. Some investigations into this phenomenon have considered whether this erroneous cleavage phenomenon could be the cause or effect of aneuploidy within the cell [15]. Since the first reports of this phenomenon, the nomenclature of this common example of early erroneous cell division has been proposed in an expert panel publication. An aberrant cleavage from a single cell directly to three daughter cells has been defined as trichotomous mitosis. This can be distinguished from "rapid" cleavages, which appear as an accelerated division event within 5 hours of the previous cell division [12]. The hypotheses of Leese et al., that preimplantation embryos that are "quiet" metabolically have greater viability than those that are not, have recently been revisited using retrospective and prospective data on metabolic and kinetic activity of preimplantation embryo development. The group considered that there may be optimal ranges that may influence embryogenesis. They proposed that these may be a "Goldilocks zone," within which embryos with maximum developmental potential can be categorized [16]. This would sit well with what is being revealed from the increasing number of published time-lapse studies. Recently, researchers have searched for novel indicators of embryo viability, only accurately recorded using time-lapse imaging. A large unpublished study at CARE Fertility Group (Nottingham, UK) examined close to 2500 blastocysts with known implantation outcomes. Unpublished logistic regression analysis demonstrated a significantly higher clinical pregnancy rate (48.9% vs. 35.9%; $p < 0.0001$) when morulae were fully compacted, with no excluded material, compared to their counterparts.

Early adopters of time-lapse and its implementation for embryo selection were Basile, Meseguer, and colleagues, who used a hierarchical approach to time-lapse algorithm development whereby embryos received a classification based primarily on reaching developmental milestones and the relative timings associated with them [17]. They reported significant differences between implanted and not implanted embryos for six early morphokinetic variables. The most significant, for implantation prediction, being the time that the embryo reached the five-cell stage (t5), and the duration of the second cell cycle (cc2). The resulting selection model also included three exclusion criteria, based on their negative association with implantation. These were rapid early division (from two to three cells), uneven blastomeres, and multinucleation at the four-cell stage. Since then, further time-lapse models have been published with variation in the time-lapse variables of significance, outcome measures, and the timings of specific developmental events [18–20].

Preimplantation Genetic Testing for Aneuploidy and Its Relationship to Time-Lapse Analysis

Preimplantation genetic testing for aneuploidy (PGT-A) is discussed in detail in a separate chapter in this book and is, like morphokinetic analysis, aimed at optimizing embryo selection by identifying embryo ploidy and enabling preferential selection of a euploid embryo for intrauterine transfer [21]. Aneuploidy is prevalent in human oocytes and embryos, and its incidence increases with maternal age. Depending on the age of the female or circumstances of the couple, more than half of their embryos are likely to be aneuploid [22]. The avoidance of selection of aneuploid embryos for transfer after IVF is a clinical imperative and the method of choice for assessing embryo ploidy currently is PGT-A, which provides a chromosome copy number of (the trophoblast cells) the blastocyst. Various technologies have been utilized, such as microarray-based comparative genomic hybridization (aCGH), single-nucleotide polymorphism (SNP) arrays or quantitative polymerase chain reaction (PCR), and next-generation sequencing (NGS), which have confirmed the high incidence of aneuploidy in human embryos with varying, but nonetheless mostly positive, reports of its efficacy [23–25].

Identification of the most viable single embryo for transfer has become increasingly important in recent years, driven by regulation (such as in the UK) and good clinical practice, to reduce the number of multiple pregnancies and births. Since 2010, with the first reported live birth after polar body biopsy and comprehensive chromosome screening, the identification of euploidy has been reported to have improved outcomes in specific circumstances, such as advanced maternal age [26–28].

PGT-A is covered in detail elsewhere; however, in brief, Anderson compared PGT-A with unscreened treatments reported in the United States in 2016 by The Society for Assisted Reproduction (SART). They found that PGT-A, in their program, outperformed the national average for live birth rate in all age groups. A recent multicenter randomized controlled trial (STAR), however, did not result in similar findings, surprising advocates of this technology, finding significant associations only for advanced maternal age [29]. The need to constantly consider alternative technologies for the assessment of both aneuploidy and overall developmental potential is therefore paramount. Despite PGT-A being considered effective at identifying euploid embryos and enhancing outcomes in some (but not all) studies, there are nonetheless limitations to this technology in association with assisted reproduction. Blastocyst biopsy—used to remove a small number of cells for assessment—requires training, specific equipment, and technical expertise, and the testing, often off-site, remains expensive and time-consuming. Furthermore, this invasive approach has raised ethical concerns and meets regulatory barriers in some countries [30].

The Possible Impact of Aneuploidy on Embryo Development

Prior to the clinical availability of time-lapse imaging, there had been reports of aneuploid embryos being delayed around the time of blastulation. In their 1998 study of mosaicism, using fluorescence *in situ* hybridization (FISH) in human blastocysts, Evsikov and Verlinsky proposed a process of selection against aneuploidy cells starting at the morula-blastocyst transition [31]. They demonstrated that human blastocysts had a significantly lower degree of mosaicism than early cleavage-stage embryos and postulated there being a threshold level of abnormal cells at which the whole embryo degenerated.

Alfarawati et al. (2011) compared blastocyst qualitative morphology with ploidy and demonstrated a weak association between blastocyst morphology and aneuploidy [32]. This group also considered embryo developmental rates and reported an insignificant trend toward aneuploid embryos showing slower progression to the most advanced blastocyst stages, and that embryos with complex aneuploidy were most delayed. This study was performed without the benefit of time-lapse technology, however, and the findings were not clinically applicable as no clear cutoff time point was given for discrimination between complex aneuploid embryos and euploid ones. The time or frequency of blastocyst morphological assessment was not discussed in that publication.

The period leading up to blastulation is a period of intense cellular metabolic activity, gene activation, rapidly increasing cell division, and differentiation. The mitotic process, resulting in cell division, is a series of complex structural rearrangements involving the kinetochore attachments to the microtubules. Cohesion molecules are essential for the precise separation of the chromosome, and they ensure correct alignment on the spindle assembly complex. Many highly specialized proteins are subject to precise gene expression control during this process [33–35].

Although the cause of a possible temporal delay in aneuploid embryos compared to their euploid counterparts may be unclear, there exist error detection and repair systems within the cells to prevent aneuploidy [36]. It is possible, therefore, that errors in individual cells at this stage of the rapidly developing embryo involve complex biochemical systems delaying karyo- and cytokinesis, which could result in the detectable delay in blastulation, particularly evident if time-lapse imaging were used. Many studies have discussed the potential value of time-lapse imaging to assess morphokinetic variables and to detect erroneous embryo development as indicators of embryo viability [5,9,12]. Several randomized controlled trials have been conducted assessing the potential benefits of morphokinetic embryo selection compared with standard methodology. A meta-analysis in 2017 reported time-lapse culture with morphokinetic embryo selection to improve pregnancy and live birth chances and reduce early pregnancy loss (Figure 7.2) [9].

Both ploidy analysis by PGT-A and morphokinetic variable analysis from time-lapse imaging are techniques that individually in some hands have demonstrated the potential to significantly improve the incidence of clinical pregnancy compared with traditional embryo culture and selection methods. Therefore, by comparison of the morphokinetics of euploid and aneuploid embryos over the preimplantation cleavage period, the key question arises regarding whether morphokinetics of euploid embryos differ from those of aneuploidy embryos, and whether there could be synergies between these technologies in ART.

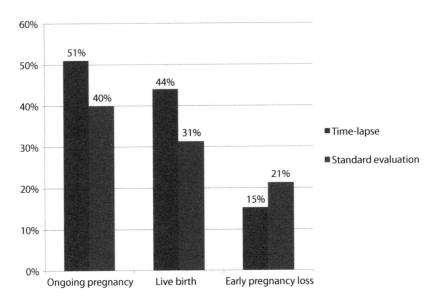

FIGURE 7.2   Summary of clinical results from meta-analysis comparing time-lapse and standard incubation and selection. (Adapted from Pribenszky et al. *Reprod Biomed Online*. Nov 1, 2017;35[5]:511–20.)

Is There an Association between Embryo Ploidy and Morphokinetics?

The first time-lapse report of an association between early human embryo development and ploidy was in 2012. Chavez and colleagues demonstrated that early cleavage events, up to the four-cell stage, were tightly clustered by timing in euploid human embryos, whereas those of aneuploid embryos were more diverse [37]. In this study, only 30% of aneuploid embryos displayed timings similar to the euploid cohort. This group used a small dataset to predict embryonic euploidy with 100% sensitivity and 66% specificity. A larger study by Basile, analyzing the chromosomal content of 504 embryos by blastomere biopsy on day 3, and aCGH, proposed a logistic regression-derived hierarchical model to subdivide embryos into four categories (A to D) according to expected risk of aneuploidy [38]. The algorithms consisted of the two morphokinetic variables, the time interval between 2 and 5 cells (>20.5 hours), and the duration of the third cleavage cycle (t5-t3) (11–18 hours). Embryos were categorized according to whether they developed within the ranges, and use of this model resulted in a significant decrease in the percentage of normal embryos with each decreasing category (A, 35.9%; B, 26.4%; C, 12.1%; and D, 9.8%; p < 0.001).

Early adopters of time-lapse for clinical IVF, Campbell and colleagues, considered whether there was a difference in the morphokinetics of euploid and aneuploid embryos by comparing data from blastocysts that had undergone PGT-A [18]. This work did not identify any early morphokinetic markers associated with ploidy, as Chavez had done and Basile went on to do. However, from the more than 20 variables compared, Campbell's group detected significant periblastulation delays in aneuploid embryos, compared with sibling euploid counterparts at the start of compaction (tSC), start of blastulation (tSB), and to the full blastocyst stage (tB). The authors then devised an aneuploidy risk classification model based on their findings, based on the two most significant morphokinetic variables (Table 7.1).

The clinical effectiveness of this model was retrospectively evaluated for the potential impact on unselected IVF patients. Following the transfer of 88 blastocysts, embryo fate up to live birth was compared according to calculated aneuploidy risk classes (low, medium, high). A significant difference was seen for implantation and live birth ratios between embryos classified with low and medium risk for aneuploidy, with relative increases of 74% and 56% for embryos within the low risk class compared to overall ratios for fetal heartbeat and live birth, respectively [40]. This study demonstrated, albeit on a small scale, the clinical relevance of such aneuploidy risk classification and introduced a novel, noninvasive method of embryo selection to yield higher implantation and live birth rates. This model was

TABLE 7.1

The Campbell Time-Lapse–Derived Model for the Classification of Ploidy with Associated Probabilities of Aneuploidy

Aneuploidy Risk Class		N	Probability
Low	tB < 122.9 hours & tSB < 96.2 hours	36	0.37
Medium	tB < 122.9 hours & tSB ≥ 96.2 hours	49	0.69
High	tB ≥ 122.9 hours	12	0.97
All		97	0.61

further successfully validated on larger and independent data from 27 clinics in relation to implantation outcome [41].

There was some criticism of this aneuploidy risk classification model by Ottolini et al., who proposed that the delays observed in the aneuploid cohort were not the result of aneuploidy, but rather associated with maternal age [42]. Campbell et al., however, published further analyses in response, which described how age alone could not account for the different proportions of euploid embryos with advancing maternal age, and suggested that embryo ploidy is a key factor controlling human embryo morphokinetics [40].

Several time-lapse studies have since also reported pericompaction and blastulation delays in aneuploidy, or embryos with low implantation potential, compared with euploid embryos, or those with high implantation potential. Minasi and colleagues, assessing a large cohort of 1730 blastocysts, asked whether there were correlations among ploidy status, morphology, and time-lapse kinetics. They reported that euploid blastocysts exhibited higher morphological quality inner cell mass and trophectoderm, and a shorter time to start blastulation, expansion, and hatching compared with aneuploid ones [43]. More recently, Mumusoglu and colleagues, using a clustered data analysis, reported a low to moderate ability to predict euploidy when patient-related factors and ovarian stimulation were considered. They reported a small number of late morphokinetic variables to be significantly different when comparing euploid and aneuploid embryo development. Later-stage delays from t9 and through to expanded blastocyst stage were reported in the aneuploid cohort [44].

Time-lapse studies considering and comparing the morphokinetics of euploid and aneuploid embryos are heterogeneic in their design and approach. However, most have not identified an association between early cleavage stage morphokinetic markers and ploidy, suggesting that euploid and aneuploid embryos develop similarly up until around the time of compaction, or around the maternal to zygotic genomic transition.

A systematic review in 2018, asking whether time-lapse parameters predict embryo ploidy, considered 13 publications between 2012 and 2017. The review also highlighted the heterogeneity of studies published to date on this topic. The 13 studies varied in stage of embryo biopsy, clinical indications for PGT-A, embryo culture conditions, statistical approaches, and outcome measures. The authors concluded that in most studies considering ploidy and morphokinetics, the intervals between cellular cleavages were of more relevance than cleavage timings in the selection of euploid embryos. It also stated that most of the studies with biopsy conducted at the blastocyst stage reported significant differences between the morphokinetics of aneuploid and euploid embryos at later (periblastulation) stages and did not find early parameters as predictors of embryo ploidy [45]. However, durations between morphokinetic variables were not comprehensively compared by all researchers. The systematic review concluded that more large-scale studies are needed to fully elucidate the putative association between ploidy and morphokinetic parameters. Further publications have since supported, and rejected, the overall findings of this review. Desai et al. assessed 767 biopsied blastocysts and reported that the presence of two or more dysmorphisms was associated with an overall lower euploidy rate, and that ploidy status correlated significantly with starting blastulation (tSB), starting expansion (tEB) and the tEB to tSB interval [46]. Zhang et al., however, did not find any morphokinetic variables to be associated with ploidy but did report that a combination of PGT-A and time-lapse monitoring improved implantation rate and ongoing pregnancy rate for PGT-A [47] (Table 7.2).

Whether pre-embryonic genome activation events, such as cleavage morphokinetics prior to the eight-cell stage, or later morphokinetic information representing the activated embryonic genome will give the most reliable selection criteria needs further study. Most of the earlier time-lapse publications focused on events up to the five-cell stage, and as a prognosticator for blastulation, or implantation, rather than live

TABLE 7.2

Summary of Studies Assessing the Relevance of Morphokinetic Variables to Predict Embryo Ploidy

First Author and Year of Publication	Time-Lapse Embryo Assessment Period	Morphokinetic Variables Associated with Ploidy Status (for Definitions See Figure 7.1)	Evidence for Potential Morphokinetic Markers of Embryo Ploidy?
Chavez et al. 2012 [37]	Early cleavage stage	cc2, s2	✓
Basile et al. 2014 [17]	Early cleavage stage	t5-t2, t5, cc3	✓
Chawla et al. 2015 [48]	Early cleavage stage	t5-t2, cc3	✓
Nogales et al. 2017 [49]	Early cleavage stage	t5-t2, t3	✓ (high risk aneuploidies)
Campbell et al. 2013 [18]	Blastocyst stage	tSC, tSB, tB	✓
Kramer et al. 2014 [50]	Blastocyst stage	None found	✗
Yang et al. 2014 [51]	Blastocyst stage	None found	✗
Rienzi et al. 2015 [52]	Blastocyst stage	None found	✗
Minasi et al. 2016 [43]	Blastocyst stage	tSB, tB, tEB, tHB	✓
Patel et al. 2016 [53]	Blastocyst stage	t5-t2, cc3	✓
Mumusoglu et al. 2017 [44]	Blastocyst stage	t9, tM, tSB, tB, tEB	✓
Desai et al. 2018 [46]	Blastocyst stage	>/=2 early stage dysmorphisms tSB, tEB, tEB-tSB	✓
Zhang et al. 2017 [47]	Blastocyst stage	None found	✗

birth [54]. While it is recognized that maternal effects may mitigate against the survival of a potentially viable embryo, and not least because aneuploidy is the largest single cause of failure, live birth outcome, in relation to morphokinetics as a selection tool, is considered the gold standard. While early time-lapse markers may be easier and therefore more objectively interpreted and assessed during annotation (or automated image analysis), they may not be as reliably representative of onward embryo development and potential following activation of the embryonic genome as later morphokinetic variables. This area of clinical research is challenging, not only due to the heterogeneity of patient populations and clinical approaches, but also because embryo ploidy is not binary, and mosaicism exists within the human embryo. Furthermore, there is increasing evidence to suggest that laboratory factors, such as humidity, culture media, or oxygen tension, could impact embryo aneuploidy [55].

Practical Benefits of Combining Time-Lapse Analysis with PGT-A

In jurisdictions where PGT-A is permissible and performed, the use of time-lapse imaging may complement this treatment, both practically and clinically. Use of a time-lapse incubation system minimizes the need to remove the embryo culture dish from the protected and controlled incubation environment. This has general advantages but for PGT-A, time-lapse can add particular value. Continuous embryo monitoring provides the embryologist preparing to undertake the trophectoderm biopsy procedure with more information about the relative developmental stages of the cohort of embryos in order to set and optimize the timing of this technically challenging microsurgical procedure. Without the facility of time-lapse imaging, the embryologist would be required to remove the culture dish from the incubator in order to assess the blastocysts and their suitability for biopsy, with little or no knowledge of where they actually are in the process of development—expansion or contraction, for example. This information may also be helpful to set patient expectations on the quality and number of embryos available. In addition, this morphokinetic information in experienced hands could be utilized to prioritize blastocysts for biopsy if the number was restricted due to capacity or cost. There is also a case for ranking euploid embryos for transfer using morphokinetic information, particularly where validated algorithms are applied, when patients are fortunate to have multiple euploids available (Figure 7.3) [47].

The impact for the IVF patient of incorporating time-lapse monitoring of embryo development goes beyond clinical outcome. The additional information provided to patients by IVF professionals regarding

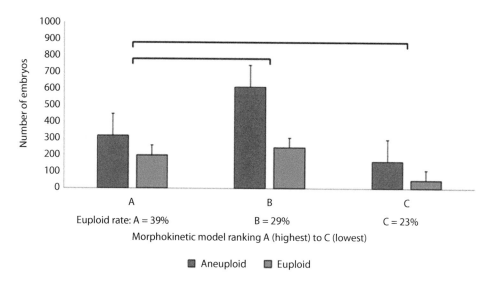

FIGURE 7.3 CARE Fertility unpublished data demonstrating that top morphokinetic grade (A) blastocysts are significantly more likely to be euploid than lower grades (B and C).

their embryos' developmental patterns and timings is more informative than standard methodology, and being able to see the images generated from this technology may enhance patient understanding and acceptance of their subfertility. Patient feedback has indicated that time-lapse technology positively aids their understanding of events in the embryology laboratory. When asked, 82% of patients reported that they agreed or strongly agreed with the statement "The use of time-lapse monitoring has improved our understanding of what happens within the IVF laboratory" (unpublished CARE fertility data, n = 363 patients) (Figure 7.4). The ability to download and view the video of their transferred embryo's first few days of development is also very well received.

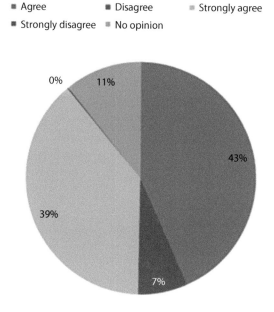

FIGURE 7.4 Pie chart to show patient feedback regarding the use of time-lapse in their IVF treatment.

Summary

Within this rapidly progressing and promising area of reproductive medicine, practitioners working with time-lapse imaging have an additional and increasingly reliable tool for noninvasively studying the human preimplantation embryo, and importantly, for improving embryo selection [9]. Despite it making practical and scientific sense to utilize this technology, which without intervention enables the collection of vast image and kinetic data for analysis alongside clinical outcomes, time-lapse imaging is considered new and unproven, and there are calls for more large-scale randomized controlled trials [56]. One of the main challenges with such trials is the differing clinical, laboratory, and embryo selection practice, which may introduce skew and affect reliability of the findings. Several large fertility clinic groups have published their own positive experiences using time-lapse and have developed selection algorithms that have been validated in-house and are in clinical use, as well as commercially available generic algorithms available through time-lapse device manufacturers [57,58].

Time-lapse technology, also in conjunction with PGT-A, has the potential to provide continuously improving embryo selection algorithms which could consider numerous criteria, resulting in algorithms defined for a range of varying circumstances, from individual patient criteria to generalized laboratory conditions. In time, the optimal ranges for defined dynamic events such as those directly associated with the "normal," or euploid, cell cycle, may be elucidated and further novel morphokinetic markers of embryo viability identified [59].

Arguably, the ultimate embryo selection tool will be reliable, reproducible, cost-effective, proven, noninvasive, and have direct clinical relevance. The most widely used approach for embryo selection that meets some but not all of these criteria is based on morphological parameters. However, this routine practice is considered somewhat limited by subjectivity. IVF professionals continually search for alternative or complementary technologies to enable improved embryo selection and, given that embryo ploidy is critical to successful outcomes, selection for euploidy is increasingly sought. The most reliable method for selection of euploid embryos in clinical use today is PGT-A. Several studies using time-lapse imaging *in vitro* have looked at the precise patterns and timings of preimplantation embryo development in relation to embryo ploidy and studied whether aneuploid and euploid embryos have different morphokinetic profiles. As a result, morphokinetic profiling has been proposed as a method to increase the probability of selecting chromosomally normal embryos noninvasively, and also to classify an embryo's risk of aneuploidy.

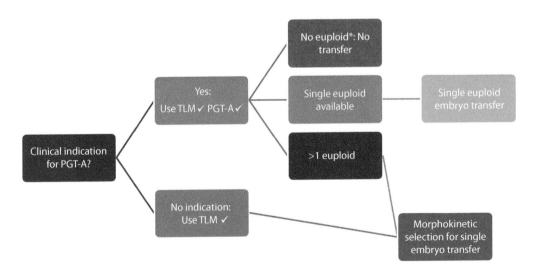

FIGURE 7.5   Proposed strategy incorporating PGT-A and time-lapse monitoring (TLM) in ART. *Some circumstances may warrant mosaic embryo transfers.

Time-lapse imaging is unlikely to ever be as absolute at elucidating ploidy from biopsied cells, or perhaps even by noninvasive PGT-A, but it is an important tool, which when utilized with precision and consistency has been reported to enhance the chances of selecting an embryo from a cohort most likely to result in a live birth following IVF by noninvasive means [39]. It may also prove to be a useful tool for ranking or prioritizing embryos for PGT-A, and for assisting in setting patient expectations, or for selecting between euploid embryos. While euploidy is a requirement for optimal healthy live birth outcome, there are many additional factors necessary within the embryo itself, and maternally, to ensure successful outcomes in ART, and it is expected that time-lapse imaging, among other viability embryo assessment methods, will increasingly be used in ART settings in combination with PGT-A (Figure 7.5).

REFERENCES

1. Gardner DK, Meseguer M, Rubio C, Treff NR. Diagnosis of human preimplantation embryo viability. *Hum Reprod Update*. 2015;21:727–47.
2. Alpha Scientists in Reproductive Medicine and ESHRE Special Interest Group of Embryology. The Istanbul consensus workshop on embryo assessment: Proceedings of an expert meeting. *Hum Reprod*. 2011;26:1270–83.
3. Alpha Scientists in Reproductive Medicine and ESHRE Special Interest Group of Embryology. The Istanbul consensus workshop on embryo assessment: Proceedings of an expert meeting. *Reprod Biomed Online*. 2011;22:632–46.
4. Cutting R et al. Elective single embryo transfer for practice. British Fertility Society and Association of Clinical Embryologists. *Hum Fertility*. 2008;11:131–46.
5. Meseguer M et al. Embryo Incubation and selection in a time-lapse monitoring system improves pregnancy outcome compared with a standard incubator: A retrospective cohort study. *Fertil Steril*. 2012;98:1481–9.
6. Rubio I et al. Limited implantation success of direct-cleaved human zygotes: A time-lapse study. *Fertil Steril*. 2012;98:1458–63.
7. Meseguer M et al. The use of morphokinetics as a predictor of embryo implantation. *Human Reprod*. 2011:26(10);2658–71.
8. Chamayou S et al. The use of morphokinetic parameters to select all embryos with full capacity to implant. *J Assist Reprod Genet*. 2013;30:703–10.
9. Pribenszky C, Nilselid AM, Montag M. Time-lapse culture with morphokinetic embryo selection improves pregnancy and live birth chances and reduces early pregnancy loss: A meta-analysis. *Reprod Biomed Online*. Nov 1, 2017;35(5):511–20.
10. Campbell A. Noninvasive techniques: Embryo selection by time lapse imaging. In: Montag M, ed. *A Practical Guide to Selecting Gametes and Embryos*. Boca Raton, FL: CRC Press; 2014:177–89.
11. Sundvall L, Ingerslev HJ, Breth Knudsen U, Kirkegaard K. Inter- and intra-observer variability of time-lapse annotations. *Human Reprod*. Sep 26, 2013;28(12):3215–21.
12. Ciray HN et al. Proposed guidelines on the nomenclature and annotation of dynamic human embryo monitoring by a time-lapse user group. *Human Reprod*. Oct 24, 2014;29(12):2650–60.
13. Barrie A, Homburg R, McDowell G, Brown J, Kingsland C, Troup S. Examining the efficacy of six published time-lapse imaging embryo selection algorithms to predict implantation to demonstrate the need for the development of specific, in-house morphokinetic selection algorithms. *Fertil Steril*. Mar 1, 2017;107(3):613–21.
14. Tran D, Cooke S, Illingworth PJ, Gardner DK. Deep learning as a predictive tool for fetal heart pregnancy following time-lapse incubation and blastocyst transfer. *Human Reprod*. May 21, 2019;34(6):1011–8.
15. Zhan Q, Ye Z, Clarke R, Rosenwaks Z, Zaninovic N. Direct unequal cleavages: Embryo developmental competence, genetic constitution and clinical outcome. *PLOS ONE*. Dec 1, 2016;11(12):e0166398.
16. Leese HJ, Guerif F, Allgar V, Brison DR, Lundin K, Sturmey RG. Biological optimization, the Goldilocks principle, and how much is *lagom* in the preimplantation embryo. *Mol Reprod Dev*. Sep, 2016;83(9):748–54.
17. Basile N et al. The use of morphokinetics as a predictor of implantation: A multicentric study to define and validate an algorithm for embryo selection. *Human Reprod*. Dec 19, 2014;30(2):276–83.
18. Campbell A et al. Modelling a risk classification of aneuploidy in human embryos using non-invasive morphokinetics. *Reprod Biomed Online*. 2013;26(5):477–85.

19. Motato Y, de los Santos MJ, Escriba MJ, Ruiz BA, Remohí J, Meseguer M. Morphokinetic analysis and embryonic prediction for blastocyst formation through an integrated time-lapse system. *Fertil Steril.* Feb 1, 2016;105(2):376–84.

20. Conaghan J et al. Improving embryo selection using a computer-automated time-lapse image analysis test plus day 3 morphology: Results from a prospective multicenter trial. *Fertil Steril.* Aug 1, 2013;100(2):412–9.

21. Fishel S et al. Assessment of 19,803 paired chromosomes and clinical outcome from first 150 cycles using array CGH of the first polar body for embryo selection and transfer. *J Fertiliz In Vitro.* 2011;1:1.

22. Fragouli E, Wells D. Aneuploidy in the human blastocyst. *Cytogenet Genome Res.* 2011;133(2–4):149–59.

23. Fragouli E, Wells D, Whalley KM, Mills JA, Faed MJ, Delhanty JD. Increased susceptibility to maternal aneuploidy demonstrated by comparative genomic hybridization analysis of human MII oocytes and first polar bodies. *Cytogenet Genome Res.* 2006;114(1):30–8.

24. Munné S, Lee A, Rosenwaks Z, Grifo J, Cohen J. Fertilization and early embryology: Diagnosis of major chromosome aneuploidies in human preimplantation embryos. *Human Reprod.* Dec 1, 1993;8(12):2185–91.

25. Yang Z et al. Selection of single blastocysts for fresh transfer via standard morphology assessment alone and with array CGH for good prognosis IVF patients: Results from a randomized pilot study. *Mol Cytogenet.* 2012;5:24.

26. Fishel S et al. Live birth after polar body array CGH prediction of embryo ploidy following IVF – the future of IVF? *Fertil Steril.* 2010;93:1006.e7–1006.e10

27. Stevens J, Rawlins M, Janesch A, Treff N, Schoolcraft WB, Katz-Jaffe MG. Time lapse observation of embryo development identifies later stage morphology based parameters associated with blastocyst quality but not chromosome constitution. *Fertil Steril.* Sep 1, 2012;98(3):S30.

28. Anderson RE, Whitney JB, Schiewe MC. Clinical benefits of preimplantation genetic testing for aneuploidy (PGT-A) for all *in vitro* fertilization treatment cycles. *Eur J Med Genet.* Feb, 2020;632(2):103731.

29. Munné S et al. Preimplantation genetic testing for aneuploidy: A pragmatic, multicenter randomized clinical trial of single frozen euploid embryo transfer versus selection by morphology alone. *Reprod Biomed Online.* Apr 1, 2019;38:e9.

30. Harper J et al. ESHG, ESHRE, EuroGentest2. Current issues in medically assisted reproduction and genetics in Europe: Research, clinical practice, ethics, legal issues and policy. *Hum Reprod.* 2014;29:1603–9.

31. Evsikov S, Verlinsky Y. Mosaicism in the inner cell mass of human blastocysts. *Hum Reprod.* 1998;13(11):3151–5

32. Alfarawati S et al. The relationship between blastocyst morphology, chromosomal abnormality and embryo gender. *Fertil Steril.* 2011;95:520–4.

33. Gonen S et al. The structure of purified kinetochores reveals multiple microtubule-attachment sites. *Nat Struct Mol Biol.* Sep 2012;19(9):925.

34. Clift D, Marston AL. The role of shugoshin in meiotic chromosome segregation. *Cytogenet Genome Res.* 2011;133(2–4):234–42.

35. Vogt E, Kirsch-Volders M, Parry J, Eichenlaub-Ritter U. Spindle formation, chromosome segregation and the spindle checkpoint in mammalian oocytes and susceptibility to meiotic error. *Mutat Res.* Mar 12, 2008;651(1–2):14–29.

36. Nasmyth K and Haering CH. Cohesin: Its roles and mechanisms. *Annu Rev Genet.* 2009;43:525–58.

37. Chavez SL et al. Dynamic blastomere behaviour reflects human embryo ploidy by the four-cell stage. *Nature Comms.* 2012;3:1251. DOI: 10.1038

38. Basile N et al. Increasing the probability of selecting chromosomally normal embryos by time-lapse morphokinetics analysis. *Fertil Steril.* Mar 1, 2014;101(3):699–704.

39. Fishel S et al. Evolution of embryo selection for IVF from subjective morphology assessment to objective time-lapse algorithms improves chance of live birth. *Reprod Biomed Online.* Oct 2020;40(1):61–70.

40. Campbell A et al. Retrospective analysis of outcomes after IVF using an aneuploidy risk model derived from time-lapse monitoring without PGS. *Reprod Biomed Online.* 2013;27:140–6

41. Campbell A, Fishel S, Laegdsmand M. Aneuploidy is a key causal factor of delays in blastulation: Author response to 'A cautionary note against aneuploidy risk assessment using time-lapse imaging'. *Reprod Biomed Online.* Mar 1, 2014;28(3):279–83.

42. Ottolini C, Rienzi L, Capalbo A. A cautionary note against embryo aneuploidy risk assessment using time-lapse imaging. *Reprod Biomed Online.* Mar 1, 2014;28(3):273–5.

43. Minasi MG et al. Correlation between aneuploidy, standard morphology evaluation and morphokinetic development in 1730 biopsied blastocysts: A consecutive case series study. *Human Reprod.* Sep 17, 2016;31(10):2245–54.

44. Mumusoglu S et al. Time-lapse morphokinetic assessment has low to moderate ability to predict euploidy when patient- and ovarian stimulation-related factors are taken into account with the use of clustered data analysis. *Fertil Steril.* Feb 1, 2017;107(2):413–21.

45. Reignier A et al. Can time-lapse parameters predict embryo ploidy? A systematic review. *Reprod Biomed Online.* 2018:26;380–7.

46. Desai N, Goldberg JM, Austin C, Falcone T. Are cleavage anomalies, multinucleation, or specific cell cycle kinetics observed with time-lapse imaging predictive of embryo developmental capacity or ploidy? *Fertil Steril.* Apr 1, 2018;109(4):665–74.

47. Zhang J et al. Morphokinetic parameters from a time-lapse monitoring system cannot accurately predict the ploidy of embryos. *J Assist Reprod Genet.* Sep 1, 2017;34(9):1173–8.

48. Chawla M et al. Morphokinetic analysis of cleavage stage embryos and its relationship to aneuploidy in a retrospective time-lapse imaging study. *J Assist Reprod Genet.* Jan 1, 2015;32(1):69–75.

49. Nogales MD et al. Type of chromosome abnormality affects embryo morphology dynamics. *Fertil Steril.* Jan 1, 2017;107(1):229–35.

50. Kramer YG et al. Assessing morphokinetic parameters via time lapse microscopy (TLM) to predict euploidy: Are aneuploidy risk classification models universal? *J Assist Reprod Genet.* Sep 1, 2014;31(9):1231–42.

51. Yang Z et al. Selection of competent blastocysts for transfer by combining time-lapse monitoring and array CGH testing for patients undergoing preimplantation genetic screening: A prospective study with sibling oocytes. *BMC Med Genomics.* Dec 2014;7(1):38.

52. Rienzi L et al. No evidence of association between blastocyst aneuploidy and morphokinetic assessment in a selected population of poor-prognosis patients: A longitudinal cohort study. *Reprod Biomed Online.* Jan 1, 2015;30(1):57–66.

53. Patel DV, Shah PB, Kotdawala AP, Herrero J, Rubio I, Banker MR. Morphokinetic behavior of euploid and aneuploid embryos analyzed by time-lapse in embryoscope. *J Hum Reprod Sci.* Apr 2016;9(2):112.

54. Wong CC et al. Non-invasive imaging of human embryos before embryonic genome activation predicts development to the blastocyst stage. *Nat Biotechnol.* Oct 2010;28(10):1115–21.

55. Swain JE. Controversies in ART: Can the IVF laboratory influence preimplantation embryo aneuploidy? *Reprod Biomed Online.* Jun 25, 2019.

56. Armstrong S, Bhide P, Jordan V, Pacey A, Farquhar C. Time-lapse systems for ART. *Reprod Biomed Online.* Mar 1, 2018;36:288–9.

57. Fishel S et al. Time-lapse imaging algorithms rank human preimplantation embryos according to the probability of live birth. *Reprod Biomed Online.* Sep 1, 2018;37(3):304–13.

58. Peterson BM, Boel M, Montag M. Development of a generally applicable morphokinetic algorithm capable of predicting the implantation potential of embryos transferred on day 3. *Hum Reprod.* 2016:31;2231–44.

59. Gallego RD, Remohí J, Meseguer M. Time-lapse imaging: The state of the art. *Biol Reprod.* Feb 27, 2019.

60. Campbell A. Time-lapse, the cell cycle, distribution of morphokinetic timings and known implantation data. Chapter 3, in *Atlas of Time Lapse Embryology*, Boca Raton, FL; CRC Press, 2015.

8

Mosaicism Mechanisms in Preimplantation Embryos

Maurizio Poli and Antonio Capalbo

CONTENTS

Introduction

Mosaicism is defined as the presence of two or more genotypically different cell lines in a given organism, embryo, or cell line. Uniform aneuploidies mostly derive from aberrant meiotic processes [1–3]. However, embryo mosaicism can originate from mitotic segregation errors in post-zygotic developmental stages of a euploid or aneuploid conceptus [4].

Mosaicism is commonly reported in the literature as being present in less than 2% of prenatal specimens (i.e., through amniocentesis or chorionic villus sampling [CVS]). In sharp contrast, it has been reported in up to 73% of cleavage-stage preimplantation embryos [5]. Due to this alleged high incidence, mosaicism has recently attracted particular attention from the scientific community in relation to its impact on embryo viability and reproductive outcome in *in vitro* fertilization (IVF) cycles with preimplantation genetic testing for aneuploidies (PGT-A). The transition between array-based to next-generation sequencing (NGS)-based technologies has marked a radical change in this field, where the technically higher sensitivity toward chromosome copy number variations has theoretically provided improved investigative tools for mosaicism status in trophectoderm (TE) biopsies. This chapter aims at providing the basic theoretical knowledge of processes giving rise to embryo mosaicism, discussing the latest studies on the subject, and providing a logic framework for management of embryo mosaicism in clinical contexts.

Classes of Mosaicism

In assisted reproduction technology (ART), embryos showing chromosomal heterogeneity are commonly defined as "mosaic." Embryonic mosaicism can be widely classified in three main categories with distinct chromosomal characteristics [6] (Figure 8.1, column F).

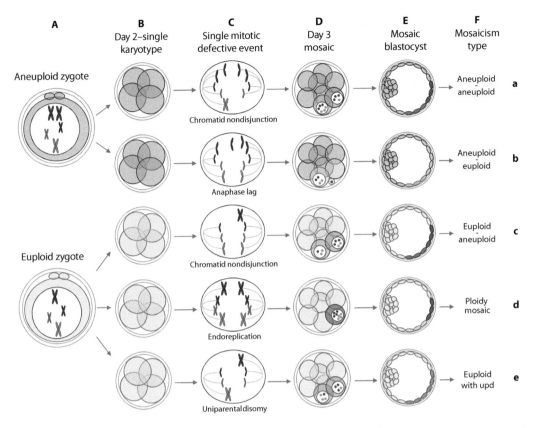

FIGURE 8.1 Examples of mosaicism progression across embryo developmental stages. Column A: Aneuploid (*purple*) and Euploid (*green*) zygotes. Column B: Day-2 embryos. Column C: Zoom-in of cellular nucleus: examples of the most common mitotic errors. Column D: Effect of defective mitotic event on embryo's cellular composition. In *purple* aneuploid cells with primary karyotype, in *red* and *blue* aneuploid cells with secondary karyotype, in *green* euploid cells with primary karyotype, in *gray* cellular fragments containing lagging chromosomes, in gray with *red* and *blue* lines euploid cells with UPD. Column E: Representation of mosaic blastocyst deriving from the specific mitotic error. Column F: Mosaicism classification.

In *aneuploid-aneuploid* mosaic embryos, all cell lineages carry chromosomal defects (i.e., absence of euploid diploid cells). This type of mosaicism commonly derives from an aneuploid zygote in which a mitotic error gives rise to cell lineages carrying different chromosomal abnormalities.

In a *euploid-aneuploid* mosaic embryo, both normal and abnormal cells are present. This scenario derives from either (i) a euploid zygote undergoing an aberrant mitotic division that generates one or more defective chromosomal sets in the embryo, or (ii) a chromosomally abnormal zygote where a mitotic event corrects the original aneuploidy, rebalancing chromosomal copies and generating a euploid cell lineage. In this latter case, uniparental disomy (UPD) can ensue.

Ploidy mosaicism entails the presence of cell lineages with different ploidy levels (i.e., diploid and tetraploid) in the same embryo. This type of mosaicism mainly derives from a cell failing to divide through cytokinesis, thus retaining, e.g., double the number of chromosomes.

Chaotic mosaicism, where multiple mitotic errors are sequentially accrued, generating several abnormal cell lineages.

Mechanisms of Formation

Mechanisms of mosaicism have not yet been completely clarified, and hypothetical causal defective processes are based on theoretical modeling. Large epidemiological and molecular studies will be required to confirm current hypotheses. Nonetheless, based on estimations, the primary cause of embryonic mosaicism is chromatid nondisjunction [7]. In addition, other aberrant processes contribute to the occurrence of mosaicism, such as anaphase lag, endoreplication, and trisomy rescue (which may lead to UPD [7–9]). UPD is an abnormal condition where both chromosome copies originate from a single parent. UPD is correlated to genetic imprinting conditions (i.e., Prader-Willi and Angelman syndromes) and can be present in the absence of abnormal chromosomal copy number (Figure 8.1, column C, row e).

Chromatid nondisjunction occurs when one set of replicated chromatids paired on metaphase plate fails to migrate to opposite mitotic poles, segregating in the same daughter cell instead. This type of defective event gives rise to two new karyotypically distinct cell lineages, one carrying a trisomy and one a monosomy (Figure 8.1, column C, row a).

Anaphase lag occurs when one chromatid fails to be incorporated in the nucleus of one of the two daughter cells. In this case, one new karyotypically distinct cell lineage is formed carrying a monosomy, while the other daughter cell remains unaffected (Figure 8.1, column C, row b). Alternatively, the lagging chromosome is also incorporated in one of the daughter cells; however, it is enclosed in a micronucleus separated from the nucleus. In the case of a trisomic zygote, anaphase lag can contribute to the generation of a euploid cell lineage within an abnormal embryo, if the chromosome in excess is excluded from the nucleus (Figure 8.1, column D, row b).

Endoreplication consists of genome replication in absence of mitosis. In this case, the chromosomal content is doubled, resulting in polyploidy. This defective mechanism is at the base of ploidy mosaicism (Figure 8.1, column C, row d).

Causative factors for defective mitotic events include relaxed control of the cell cycle, aberrations of the centrosome and mitotic spindle, and defects in chromosome cohesion [6]. In addition, it has been suggested that ovarian stimulation regimens and IVF culture conditions may also promote the occurrence of mitotic errors [10]. However, these results were generated using fluorescent *in situ* hybridization (FISH), and more comprehensive, sensitive, and up-to-date technologies, in carefully designed studies, would be required to validate these findings.

Impact of Mosaicism on the Embryo

Depending on the developmental stage at which the mitotic error occurs in an embryo, the secondary karyotype will manifest in a different proportion of cells [7] (Figure 8.2). Theoretically, the stage at which the mitotic error takes place impacts the overall proportion of the embryo containing the secondary karyotype, where the earlier the error occurs, the higher the portion of the embryo is

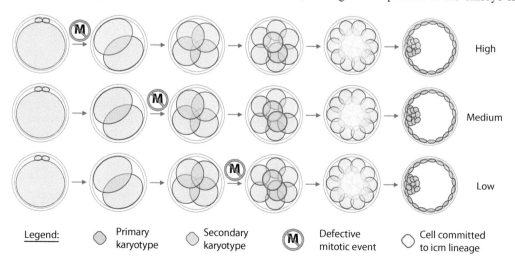

FIGURE 8.2 The proportion of embryo carrying a secondary karyotype depends on embryo developmental stage at the time of defective mitotic event.

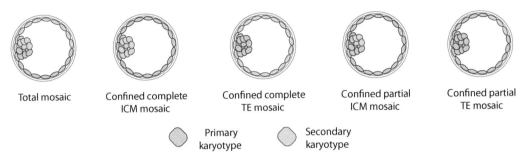

FIGURE 8.3 Simplified representation of mosaic embryo classification based on involvement of differentiating tissues.

affected. However, certain chromosomal defects (especially if complex) may cause the arrest of the cell cycle in the affected cell, thus avoiding its proportional contribution to the ensuing embryo. In addition, depending on the cell lineage commitment undertaken by the cells affected by the mitotic error, mosaicism can be distributed throughout the embryo or confined to a certain tissue (e.g., inner cell mass [ICM], TE) [11]. As a result, the fewer the cells present in the embryo at the time the defective mitotic event occurs, the higher the chance that mosaicism will involve both embryonic and extra-embryonic tissues (Figure 8.2).

Early embryonic cells maintain pluripotency, thus being able to differentiate in all cell lineages. *In vivo*, following multiple rounds of cell division, embryonic cells enter irreversible pathways of differentiation, which will be maintained in subsequent divisions [12]. If the defective mitotic event occurs after a certain differentiation pathway is undertaken, only that cell lineage or part of that tissue will be affected (Figure 8.2). Lineage commitment of cells carrying secondary karyotypes has significant impact on the type of mosaicism affecting the embryo. For instance, when both main embryo cell lineages (e.g., ICM, TE) are composed of primary and secondary karyotypes (i.e., defective mitotic event occurring at a very early developmental stage), the embryo will show *total mosaicism* (Figure 8.3a). Alternatively, if the defective mitotic event occurs at the earliest stage of cell lineage commitment, the secondary karyotype will be equally represented in all cells composing the specific tissue and all the cells deriving from downstream differentiation processes (*confined complete TE/ICM mosaicism*) (Figure 8.3b, c). If the defective mitotic event occurs in a differentiated cell after several divisions, the secondary karyotype will be present only in part of the tissue and in some of the subsequently differentiating tissues (i.e., *confined partial ICM mosaicism, confined partial TE mosaicism*) (Figure 8.3d, e). This latest case is at the base of organ-specific mosaicism like confined placental mosaicism and germinal mosaicism.

How Is Mosaicism Detected?

The first evidence of mosaicism in human embryos was produced using FISH [13]. In this case, several blastomeres from a cleavage-stage embryo were analyzed and discordant numbers of sexual chromosomes identified. With the concomitant development of comprehensive chromosome screening techniques for PGT (i.e., array comparative genomic hybridization [aCGH], array single nucleotide polymorphism [aSNP], quantitative polymerase chain reaction [qPCR]) alongside blastocyst culture and biopsy, direct single-cell analysis was abandoned. Indeed, the karyotype of a group of cells was assessed indirectly by comparing the signal produced by amplified and fluorescently labeled DNA of the test sample with a control. The fluorescence signal was transformed into data points plotted on a scale representing the length of each chromosome. If the signal for a specific chromosome showed a consistent log2 increment compared to the control, this determined the presence of trisomy. If the signal showed a consistent log2 reduction compared with the control, monosomy was diagnosed. Using these methodologies, the detection of mosaicism was performed by identification of intermediate log2 values [14,15]. With the introduction of NGS, the increased analytical resolution and diagnostic sensitivity have made it possible to discriminate with more precision the subtle chromosomal variations in PGT-A analyses (see also Chapter 3). It has been reported that NGS can discriminate proportions of karyotypically different cell mixtures as low as 20% [16].

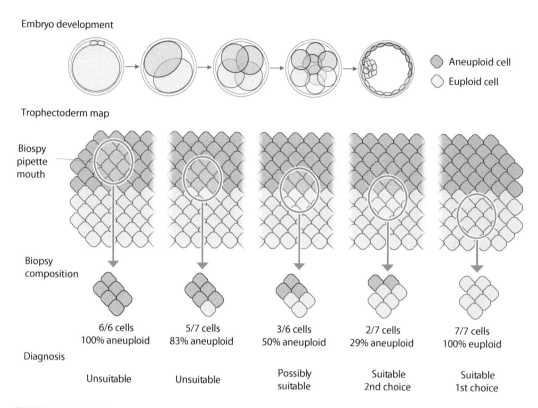

FIGURE 8.4 Visual representation of how the stochastic nature of TE biopsy can severely impact on diagnostic results and embryonic fate. A TE with the same proportion of cells carrying primary and secondary karyotypes can give a range of different diagnostic results depending on the portion of TE biopsied.

In 2016, the PGDIS position statement on PGT-A recommended that NGS diagnoses of euploid embryos with chromosome copy number variations between 20% and 80% should be considered as mosaics, below 20% should be considered fully euploid, while over 80% should be considered fully aneuploid. Unfortunately, these criteria do not take into account either biological variability across cellular specimens or the generation of technical artifacts and noise signals introduced by whole-genome amplification (WGA) prior to aCGH or NGS in low-input samples [7] (see Technical Limitations of Mosaicism Diagnosis in Cleavage and Trophectoderm Biopsies), which could result in the generation of intermediate profiles.

In addition, it is not possible to determine the primary and secondary karyotype of the embryo only based on the proportion of DNA analyzed through a single biopsy. Indeed, random cell sampling does not provide unequivocal representation of the whole embryo's karyotype, allowing stochastic processes to affect the veridicality of the diagnosis (Figure 8.4).

In support of these considerations, a recent article by Victor and colleagues reported that additional biopsies of alleged mosaic embryos did actually produce either fully euploid (both ICM and second TE biopsy), reciprocal mosaic aneuploidy, or confirm the presence of mosaicism, although at different degrees (i.e., low vs. high) [17]. By following up the transfer of 100 mosaic embryos, Victor and colleagues showed that embryos with single mosaic aneuploidy had similar implantation and fetal heartbeat outcomes to fully euploid embryos, irrespective of their level of mosaicism. This finding is in line with previous studies showing suboptimal sensitivity and specificity in mosaicism calling when biological specimens are assessed in parallel with cell line mixture models [18]. In addition, they showed that differences in clinical performance of mosaic embryos was related to the patient's age rather than level of mosaicism, suggesting that mosaic embryos were more likely to be fully aneuploid in older patients, thus highlighting the shortcomings of intermediate chromosomal levels in providing sufficient accuracy and robustness for mosaicism diagnosis.

A recent work by Popovic and colleagues re-analyzed the karyotype of outgrowths of previously biopsied human blastocysts. In their work, they showed that if mosaicism was not considered during analysis, the concordance between TE biopsy and outgrowth karyotypes was 100%, with 0% false negative and positive results, compared with an accuracy of 80% and 0% false negative and 18.5% false positive result when mosaicism was considered [19].

In 2016, Capalbo and colleagues highlighted how true evidence of chromosomal mosaicism in embryos should be collected prior to reporting it, arguing that the criteria currently used are of the lowest standards [20] (Figure 8.5). Also, profile plots resembling mosaicism can occur as a consequence of several biological

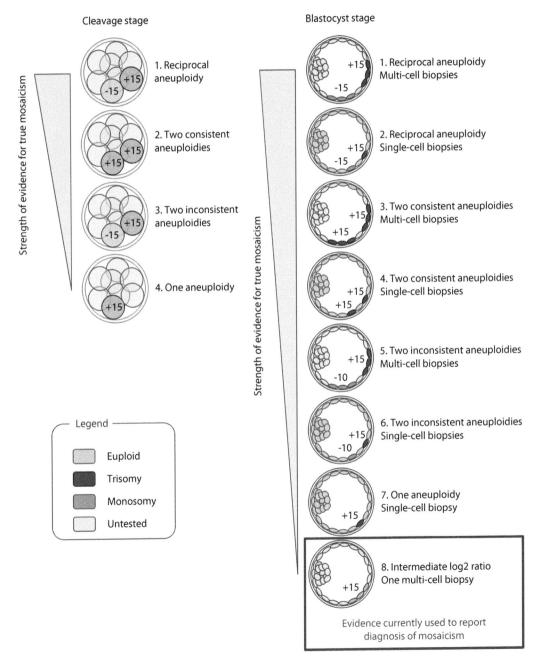

FIGURE 8.5 Model for evaluating evidence of embryonic mosaicism for diagnostic purposes. Proposed by Capalbo and colleagues. (Adapted from Capalbo A et al. *Hum Reprod.* 2016;32(3):492–8.)

phenomena occurring in the embryo (i.e., intermediate S-phase cell analysis, monosomy/trisomy in polyploidy embryo). Thus, reporting a diagnosis of mosaicism can be considered conceptually biased [21].

Nonetheless, reporting embryo mosaicism generates a course of action that often impacts the practice and outcomes of the IVF treatment. This occurrence is increased when stringency thresholds for mosaicism detection are artificially placed at minimal-maximal degrees of mosaic aneuploidy (i.e., 20%–80%). A recent web-based survey showed that almost 50% of IVF centers performing PGT and receiving details regarding mosaicism consider an embryo as mosaic when abnormal cells are expected to be present in 20% of the tested sample [22]. However, when low limits are employed, both the incidence of mosaicism detection and the overall diagnostic uncertainty increase. This means that when the thresholds used to determine the presence of mosaicism are placed as low as 20%, we will identify an increasing number of mosaic embryos, although their actual chromosomal status may be different.

Technical Limitations of Mosaicism Diagnosis in Cleavage and Trophectoderm Biopsies

Technical Errors from Cleavage-Stage Single-Cell Studies

Mosaicism rates in human preimplantation embryos at cleavage stage were found to be as high as 90% [23–26]. However, these results have been shown to be severely biased by the low sensitivity of the technique used (FISH) and the weak criteria employed for mosaicism assessment, where only one single discordant cell was sufficient to define an embryo as mosaic [7]. In fact, when individual blastomeres are analyzed by FISH, the intrinsic technical error combined with weak classification criteria can lead to misidentification of aneuploidies in cells derived from euploid embryos, suggesting the presence of mosaicism. Considering a conservative FISH positive error rate of 10% [27], the probability of identifying a false positive aneuploid cell in a uniform euploid embryo is estimated to be 40% in a 6-cell embryo $(1\text{-}0.9^6)$, 57% in an 8-cell embryo $(1\text{-}0.9^8)$, and 70% in a 10-cell embryo $(1\text{-}0.9^{10})$.

A study by Treff and colleagues showed that when cells deriving from the same embryo are analyzed in parallel with FISH and a comprehensive chromosome testing (CCT) method (e.g., SNP), mosaicism estimations can vary significantly between techniques (100% mosaicism diagnosis in FISH vs. 31% in SNP array) [27]. This consideration emphasized how technical efficiency severely impacts the perceived incidence of mosaicism in preimplantation embryos. More recent studies have also highlighted how cell cycle– related issues might contribute to a distortion of the profile plot obtained using more comprehensive molecular technologies for 24-chromosome testing of a single cell, resulting in mosaicism overestimation at the cleavage stage [28].

When the cytogenetic status of embryos at the blastocyst stage was evaluated in multiple biopsies of the same embryo using CCT, the incidence of mosaicism was found to be reduced compared to cleavage-stage embryos (5% vs. 31%, respectively, [20]. This difference in mosaicism incidence is possibly due to a higher methodological robustness and accuracy of multicellular samples from the TE compared to single blastomere analysis rather than a selective depletive mechanism of aneuploid/mosaic cells.

Technical Errors Affecting Mosaicism Detection in Blastocyst-Stage Multicellular Biopsies

By providing a higher resolution to define chromosome copy number variations (CNV) compared to previously employed methodologies (i.e., aCGH, qPCR), NGS has enabled mosaicism diagnoses based on intermediate variations of the data points related to a specific region of the genome (Figure 8.6a). Despite being more accurate, NGS-based copy number analysis is not expected to be a bias-free technology for mosaicism assessment. As in every analytical measurement, sampling is prone to technical and experimental variability. Indeed, the algorithms used to determine the ploidy status are based on the distribution of data points generated during experimental technical validation and their dispersion from mean values of reference samples. However, these thresholds aren't absolutely defined and accurate. Depending on the precision of the specific technology used, a subset of results generated from reference

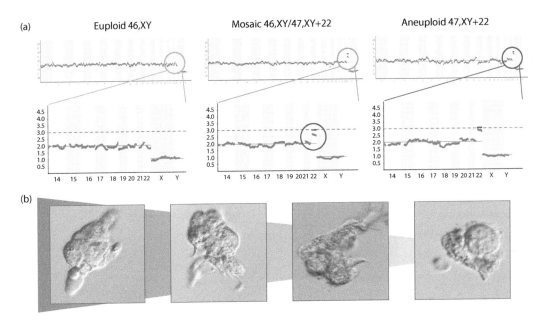

FIGURE 8.6 Technical and biological variations impacting on the reliability of mosaicism diagnoses. (a) Examples of CCT profiles of euploid, mosaic, and aneuploid TE biopsies; (b) examples of the heterogeneity of TE biopsy quality. Good to poor quality, left to right.

samples will inevitably overlap with different categories used for classification (i.e., euploid, mosaic, and aneuploid) as a result of technical variability of the method.

Hence, it should be acknowledged that a minority of normal samples can produce data above or under the thresholds used to define normal profiles and will therefore be reported as abnormal (or mosaic in this case). On the other hand, some aneuploid samples can produce intermediate copy number values lying in the mosaic range, producing a false negative (or false intermediate in this case) result.

Goodrich and colleagues recently tested the precision of NGS in discriminating the proportion of abnormal cells in a given sample. This type of approach was validated on mixtures of normal and aneuploid cell lines, where the ratio between abnormal and normal cells was gradually incremented and the accuracy in identifying CNV for the chromosomes tested was calculated. A correlation between the average chromosome copy number of the specific chromosomal aneuploidy tested and the ratio of abnormal cells was identified [18]. However, an intrinsic variability across samples and experiments was reported, showing high standard deviations and substantial overlapping across mosaicism categories. For example, sample mixtures of 33% triploid cells for chromosome 13 produced data compatible with both full euploidy and 67% aneuploid mosaicism, leading to uncertainty in the diagnostic call. Similar uncertainty was observed in all other chromosomes tested (e.g., 15, 18, and X). In practical terms, attempting to optimize specificity toward mosaicism detection (true positive calls) is possible by decreasing stringency on diagnostic call thresholds. However, this strategy inevitably results in less specificity and increased false positive diagnosis of mosaicism. Hence, threshold manipulation should be carefully assessed and cautiously employed to not lower the accuracy in uniform euploid and aneuploid embryos identification.

Furthermore, the difference in biological characteristics between clinical TE biopsies and cell samples obtained from cell lines should not be underestimated or oversimplified. Mosaicism thresholds generated in experimental settings are based on defined mixes of isolated cells from cell lines, which provide only "ideal" and stable *in vitro* experimental modeling of mosaicism. Real TE biopsies are characterized by higher variability in cellular quality and quantity compared to cell line mixture models. Thus, the application of experimentally derived thresholds to the clinical situation is challenging and prone to inherent errors, especially when they are applied to TE biopsies, which are heterogeneous in nature (Figure 8.6b).

Incidence of Mosaicism

Depending on the karyotype of the zygote (e.g., euploid, aneuploid), the defective mitotic event has different impacts on the embryo. For instance, a defective event occurring in a euploid cell always produces two aneuploid daughter cells. On the other hand, an aneuploid embryo could generate a subpopulation of euploid cells with deleterious consequences for diagnostic results. Despite the current possibility of detecting the presence of mosaicism in an embryo, it is not possible to discern the karyotype of the progenitor zygote from the chromosomal analysis of a single biopsy specimen. Unless the whole embryo is analyzed cell by cell and the chromosomal status of the progenitor zygote inferred from the percentage of cells for each karyotype, it is not possible to define the predominant karyotype in a mosaic embryo. Alternatively, the detection of reciprocal aneuploidies in two distinct biopsy specimens would allow the identification of the zygote's original karyotype. However, this approach would be very invasive for the embryo and not feasible from a clinical standpoint.

The extent to which a randomly sampled population of cells collected during biopsy is representative of the main body of the blastocyst is the main diagnostic uncertainty associated with PGT-A. For this reason, it is crucial that the incidence of mosaicism and its impact on embryo implantation and development are accurately determined, as well as any consequences embryo mosaicism may have on the pregnancy.

Incidence of mosaicism in human fetuses was reported to be lower than 0.5% [29]. When CVS testing or amniocentesis were followed up, no differences were reported in incidence of mosaicism between natural and IVF pregnancies [29,30]. These results suggest that IVF-related procedures are not an independent risk factor for the occurrence of mosaicism in preimplantation embryos. However, this evidence is in sharp contrast with the high incidence reported from PGT-A studies. It has been hypothesized that in a mosaic embryo, chromosomally abnormal cells may be selectively depleted during development, leading to an organism composed of euploid cells only [31,32]. A euploid lineage selection process was demonstrated in a murine model by Bolton and colleagues [33]. However, similar mechanisms in human embryos are still to be demonstrated. In addition, since aneuploidy in murines is not as frequent as in humans, mitotic errors in chromosome segregation had to be induced with administration of an exogenous compound (e.g., reversine). It is a possibility that the internalization of this chemical had a lethal effect on the cell, which was then depleted from the developing embryo not because of an aneuploidy self-detection mechanism but rather due to the cytotoxic effect of the compound. In addition, reversine treatment was shown to induce complex chromosomal alterations [33], instead of single aneuploidies, which are more common in human blastocysts [34]. For this reason, it is possible that the presence of complex abnormalities would result in cell cycle arrest, thus depleting aneuploid cells from the embryo. Although some of the data published suggest no preferential allocation of abnormal cells in specific cell lineages in human mosaic embryos [35], at present, no evidence about the existence of a correction/depletion mechanism of aneuploid through developmental progression has been reported. It is well documented how every chromosome can be found in an abnormal copy number (including full haploid configuration) in embryos at the blastocyst stage [7]. A large set of aneuploidies are also compatible with sustained implantation [36]. These observations suggest that a depletive mechanism targeting aneuploid cells in mosaic embryos after embryo genome activation (EGA) cannot alone explain either the significant reduction in mosaicism diagnosis in blastocyst-stage embryos compared to cleavage stage ones or the extremely low incidence of mosaicism in miscarried products of conception (POC).

Future functional studies on human models will be required to understand how abnormal cells propagate in the pre- and postimplantation window in comparison to euploid ones. Moreover, it is also possible that an abnormal mitotic event occurs in the postimplantation period leading to the generation of mosaic pregnancies from uniformly euploid preimplantation embryos and explaining part of the mosaic cases observed in prenatal diagnosis (PND) and, for example, in cases of germinal mosaicism. Accordingly, at present, the large difference between mosaicism rates reported at the preimplantation and prenatal stages appear to be unsupported by a mechanism of depletion of abnormal cells throughout development.

Impact on Treatment Outcome

The lack of convincing data on the actual developmental potential of mosaic embryos generates decisional uncertainty. In fact, by using wide thresholds for mosaicism, not only the number of embryos with an uncertain diagnosis escalates, but also the decision on how to use them becomes more difficult. Are these embryos safe to transfer? If we transferred them, would we expose our patients to an increased risk of miscarriage or abnormal conception? Or are we overcalling chromosomal abnormalities in PGT cycles? This uncertainty will magnify as the number of mosaic embryo diagnoses increases.

In an effort to help patients in this decision, genetic counseling is usually offered, which often results in the safest, although least effective, course of action: abandonment of the supposedly mosaic embryos and, when possible, embarkment on potentially unnecessary additional IVF treatments.

In a recent study by Munnè and colleagues, it is evident how abandonment of allegedly mosaic embryos is largely preferred to their transfer [37]. In this study, only 143 out of 6368 (2.2%) embryos diagnosed with some type of mosaicism were transferred to the patients, while the vast majority were discarded or left in the cryotank. Due to the large biases involved in mosaicism diagnoses discussed previously, it is probable that many of these untransferred embryos are actually fully euploid or carry a minor alteration in their karyotype. Nonetheless, the diagnosis of mosaicism has indirectly determined their ineligibility for clinical use, regardless of their true chromosomal status.

Despite the severe clinical implications and the fact that only a few retrospective studies have investigated mosaicism clinical predictive value, reporting of mosaicism has become a standard practice in many PGT laboratories. In the same study by Munnè and colleagues, embryo transfer outcomes and pregnancies derived from euploid and mosaic embryos (including complex, single, double, monosomic, trisomic, and segmental at both low mosaicism [20%–40%] and high mosaicism [>40%]) were followed up. Cumulative results from all centers involved in the study show significant difference in implantation and miscarriage rates between the two groups [37]. Conversely, a study by Fragouli and colleagues showed no statistical difference in clinical outcomes between euploid embryos and embryos displaying several types of mosaic-consistent diagnosis (implantation rate, $p = 0.1$; miscarriage rate, $p = 0.462$; Table 8.1) [38]. Another study by Spinella and colleagues where the grade of mosaicism was also considered showed that low-grade mosaicism and fully euploid embryos produced similar implantation and miscarriage rates (Table 8.1). However, high-grade mosaic embryos showed significantly reduced implantation and clinical pregnancy rates compared to low-grade mosaic embryos. Indeed, when clinical outcomes of embryos with high-grade mosaicism were included in the calculations, a decrease in clinical performance was observed in the mosaic group in terms of implantation, but not in miscarriage rates [16]. Regardless of the contrasting results in clinical performance reported by these studies, the identification of mosaicism in embryos remains equivocal. Indeed, not a single true positive confirmation of mosaicism diagnosis by POC or PND cytogenetic analysis has been reported following the transfer of a mosaic IVF embryo so far.

Unfortunately, none of these studies discuss the reasons why the allegedly mosaic embryos were selected for transfer. It can be argued that the patient population that received these embryos was not matched with the one that received euploid embryos.

Both biological and technical biases can derive from this type of population selection. For instance, it is possible that good-prognosis patients did not routinely receive mosaic embryos as they had fully euploid embryos to select from. Also, poor-prognosis patients were more likely to have fewer embryos to choose from, increasing their chance to receive mosaic embryos. In addition, aneuploid embryos could have been erroneously classified as highly mosaic embryos, biasing the composition of the group and the corresponding outcomes. Finally, when mosaic embryos were selected against, they were employed in later transfers, which are known to produce lower success rates, even in cycles not involving PGT analysis.

It follows that, in the absence of data from prospective studies, the decision of abandoning allegedly mosaic embryos in the cryotank is not the most efficient strategy to deal with the diagnosis of mosaicism, and it leads to a considerable wastage of reproductively competent embryos able to generate a healthy pregnancy.

The uncertainty surrounding the clinical implications of transferring a mosaic embryo can generate confusion in the medical and genetic counselor that not only triggers anxiety in the patient, but also

TABLE 8.1

Difference in Clinical Outcomes between Euploid Embryos and Embryos Displaying Several Types of Mosaic-Consistent Diagnosis

	Mosaic All N % (95%CI)	Euploid N % (95%CI)	p-value		N % (95%CI)	N % (95%CI)	
Munné *(all centers)*							
Implantation rate	76/143 **53.2** *(44.6–61.5)*	736/1045 **70.4** *(67.6–73.2)*	<0.001				
Miscarriage rate	19/76 **25.0** *(15.8–36.3)*	75/736 **10.2** *(8.1–12.6)*	<0.001		**Mosaic <50%**	**Euploid**	**p-value**
Fragouli							
Implantation rate	17/44 **38.6** *(24.2–54.5)*	29/51 **56.0** *(42.2–70.6)*	0.1	**Spinella** Implantation rate	22/45 **48.9** *(33.7–64.2)*	137/251 **54.6** *(48.2–60.8)*	0.519
Miscarriage rate	5/17 **29.4** *(10.3–56.0)*	5/29 **17.2** *(5.8–35.8)*	0.462	Miscarriage rate	3/22 **13.6** *(2.9–34.9)*	20/137 **14.6** *(9.1–21.6)*	1
Spinella					**Mosaic <50%**	**Mosaic >50%**	
Implantation rate	30/78 **38.5** *(27.7–50.2)*	137/251 **54.6** *(48.2–60.8)*	0.014	Implantation rate	22/45 **48.9** *(33.7–64.2)*	8/33 **24.2** *(11.9–42.3)*	0.035
Miscarriage rate	6/30 **20.0** *(7.7–38.6)*	20/137 **14.6** *(9.1–21.6)*	0.577	Miscarriage rate	3/22 **13.6** *(2.9–34.9)*	3/8 **37.5** *(8.5–75.5)*	0.300

Source: Data derived from Munné S et al. *Fertil Steril.* 2017;108(1):62–71.e8; Fragouli E et al. *Hum Genet.* 2017;136(7):805–19; Spinella F et al. *Fertil Steril.* 2018;109(1):77–83.

may occasionally have counterproductive consequences on the overall fertility treatment. These include decreased treatment cost-efficacy due to unnecessary counseling sessions, additional embryo screening tests, extra IVF treatment cycles and, most importantly, potential wastage of reproductively competent embryos. In future studies, it is thus extremely important to define the clinical positive and negative predictive values of a "mosaic-consistent" diagnosis in well-designed prospective studies.

Reporting of Mosaicism

In order to minimize the negative effects of a mosaicism diagnosis, it is crucial to define the importance of the information that is reported to the patient and ensure that its relevance is explained based on unbiased and comprehensive data. Despite the fact that in some PGT-A practices mosaicism diagnoses have a vast impact on the treatment of patients, no conclusive data on their biological and clinical consequences have yet been gathered. Until this evidence is available, it is crucial that all the previously mentioned limitations are clearly highlighted in consent forms and that the lack of robust data from prospective studies are acknowledged and thoroughly discussed in the context of reproductive and genetic counseling.

While definitive resolutions are being investigated through studies with higher statistical strength, decisional checkpoints can be employed to minimize the potential negative effects of mosaicism reporting on IVF treatments.

In conventional PGT cycles, chromosomal status is the most relevant criterion employed in deciding the embryo that should be transferred, followed by morphological score. As a first approach, the threshold's stringency to define presence of mosaicism should be tightened, maximizing the precision in detecting uniform euploid and aneuploid status and reducing diagnostic uncertainty. However, at present, intermediate copy number values consistent with mosaicism cannot be completely disregarded, and additional decisional checkpoints should be employed in the case of mosaicism diagnosis for some of the embryos tested.

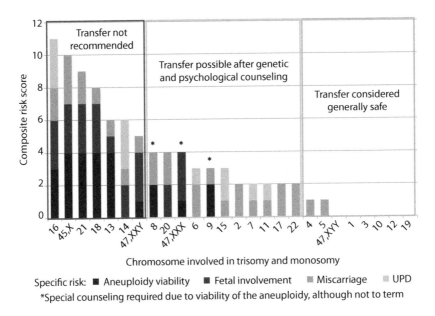

FIGURE 8.7   Mosaicism Risk-Scoring System. The Graph Takes Into Consideration (I) The Risk Of A Certain Aneuploidy To Result In Full-Term Pregnancy; (Ii) The Likelihood That A Mosaic Aneuploidy Would Involve The Fetus (*Purple*); (Iii) The Chance A Specific Chromosomal Mosaicism Would Result In Miscarriage (*Light Purple*); (Iv) The Incidence That A Uniparental Disomy Would Involve A Clinically Significant Condition In The Fetus (*Very Light Purple*). (Data from Grati FR et al. *Reprod Biomed Online.* 2018;36(4):442–9.)

In the presence of equal morphological grading, transfer priority should be given to the euploid embryo. However, in the presence of allegedly mosaic embryos with higher morphological grading compared to the available euploid embryo(s), additional criteria should be employed.

Provided that mosaicism is reported only for embryos with a ratio of aneuploid cells not lower than 30%, careful consideration should be given to the chromosomes involved in the alteration. In a recent study, Grati and colleagues analyzed over 70,000 CVS and over 3800 POCs in order to assess incidence and risk of adverse outcome in the case of mosaicism for each chromosome [4]. Taking into consideration (i) the risk of a certain aneuploidy to result in full-term pregnancy; (ii) the likelihood that a mosaic aneuploidy present in the villi would involve the fetus (and not only the placenta); (iii) the incidence that a uniparental disomy present in the villi would involve a clinically significant condition in the fetus, and (iv) the chance that a specific chromosomal mosaicism would result in miscarriage, they have produced a mosaicism risk score to help in the selection of which mosaic embryos might be eligible for transfer (Figure 8.7). This information can help clinicians and embryologists in counseling patients regarding the risks of transferring a mosaic embryo. Based on these data, the transfer of embryos showing certain types of mosaicism should be avoided because of the increased life-threating risks associated. These cases involve aneuploidies that are (i) compatible with life (i.e., mosaic trisomies for chromosomes, 21; 18; 13, and 45,X), (ii) compatible with late fetal development (i.e., mosaic trisomies for chromosome 16), (iii) associated with a high chance of deriving from uniparental disomy (i.e., mosaic trisomies for chromosome 14), and (iv) highly likely to involve the fetus (i.e., 47,XXY).

Monosomies of autosomal chromosomes are usually considered as having a less negative consequence, as they are not compatible with fetal life. This means that if a mosaic embryo carrying a monosomy were transferred, in the worst-case scenario it would fail to implant or lead to early miscarriage. On the other hand, the transfer of a mosaic embryo carrying a trisomy could also potentially result in the birth of a child with a severe chromosomal aberration. Hence, because of the lack of long-term negative consequences and potential impact on the mother's and family's well-being, the transfer of an embryo showing a mosaic profile involving an autosomic monosomy can be considered "safer" than an embryo showing a mosaic autosomic trisomy. However, it is also important to note that, if a monosomy is detected, there is a considerable chance that the reciprocal trisomic cell line may be present should the TE be rebiopsied in a different location. Thus, monosomic mosaic findings for chromosomes with important fetal involvement (listed previously), should be considered at the same risk level of trisomic mosaic ones. For all the other potentially mosaic configurations, morphological grading should be used to prioritize embryos without altered CNVs, as the use of mosaicism criteria is currently not supported by sufficient clinical evidence.

In intermediate profiles where the potential presence of mosaicism and a severe phenotype (i.e., viable aneuploidy, UPD, miscarriage, and mosaicism fetal involvement) are not strongly associated, patients should undergo detailed genetic and psychological counseling prior to embryo transfer.

Especially in these cases, genetic counseling is an integral part of the decision-making process by providing the patients unbiased information regarding the diagnostic capabilities and limitations of current PGT and the short- and long-term implications of the transfer of a mosaic embryo based on up-to-date information.

Clinical Follow-Up of Mosaic Embryos

Prenatal diagnosis is always advised in IVF treatments involving PGT. Importantly, PND is even more strongly recommended when potentially mosaic embryos are transferred due to the likely increased risk of fetal aneuploidy. In particular, amniocentesis should be preferred to other types of prenatal investigation because it includes cells deriving from the fetus and not only from extra-embryonic tissues (e.g., chorionic villi), thus minimizing the risk of detection of placenta-confined mosaicism. Extended analysis and/ or cell count of amniocytes to exclude the presence of low-level mosaicism in the fetus should also be standard practice.

Because of trophectoderm involvement in the development of the chorionic structure, CVS might not be recommendable for verifying the mosaicism status of the fetus because of the increased risk of detecting the same mosaic aneuploidy observed in PGT at the blastocyst stage. Hence, this type of result would not be advantageous in determining the true chromosomal status of the fetus.

Similarly, cell-free DNA-based (cfDNA) testing is not recommended in cases of suspected mosaicism because the fragments of DNA detected in noninvasive prenatal screening (NIPT) derive from apoptotic cells from the cytotrophoblast, hence not representing the actual fetal karyotype [39,40]. Because the amniotic fluid contains a high proportion of fetal cells, amniocentesis is the diagnostic method of choice in cases of suspected fetal mosaicism [36].

Future Perspectives for Management of Embryo Mosaicism

It has been reported how an altered chromosomal copy number can originate from both technical variation and biological phenomena other than mosaicism. Inherent inaccuracy in the methods employed for chromosome copy number estimation, as well as the inconsistency of the criteria used to define mosaicism detection, has led to an overestimation of its occurrence in IVF embryos by some genetic laboratories. Due to the potential for alternative technical and biological explanation of the result, these altered chromosomal profiles would be better reported as "profiles consistent with mosaicism" or "pro-mosaic profile," rather than as a definite diagnosis. For this reason, mosaicism should be acknowledged in the PGT consent form as a limitation of the testing methodology, as it is commonly referred to during PND (i.e., CVS and amniocentesis). Also, it should be stated that this shortcoming should not impose risks higher than IVF without PGT, considering that it will not have a major impact on clinical outcomes (as demonstrated by the low incidence observed in human blastocysts and pregnancies) and by the positive outcomes of published randomized clinical trials (RCTs) on PGT clinical effectiveness [41–43]. Also, it should be considered that, in the light of most recent evidence, avoiding mosaicism reporting might be preferable, as it improves diagnostic accuracy, drastically reducing the occurrence of false positive calls and associated clinical consequences [17,19].

It is crucial for future understanding of this important issue in reproductive medicine and genetics that the clinical outcome of mosaic embryos is monitored and properly assessed in prospective nonselection studies, unbiased by external confounding factors such as patient's prognosis and embryo morphology. By producing ultimate, uncontroversial level I evidence on this subject, clinical predictive values of new mosaicism classification schemes will improve decision-making procedures, fine-tuning PGT-A cycles and relieving patients and professionals from uncertain diagnostic outcomes.

REFERENCES

1. Hassold T, Hunt P. To err (meiotically) is human: The genesis of human aneuploidy. *Nat Rev Genet.* 2001;2(4):280–91.
2. Ottolini CS et al. Genome-wide maps of recombination and chromosome segregation in human oocytes and embryos show selection for maternal recombination rates. *Nat Genet.* 2015;47(7):727–35.
3. Capalbo A et al. Human female meiosis revised: New insights into the mechanisms of chromosome segregation and aneuploidies from advanced genomics and time-lapse imaging. *Hum Reprod Update.* 2017;23(6):706–22.
4. Grati FR et al. An evidence-based scoring system for prioritizing mosaic aneuploid embryos following preimplantation genetic screening. *Reprod Biomed Online.* 2018;36(4):442–9.
5. van Echten-Arends J et al. Chromosomal mosaicism in human preimplantation embryos: A systematic review. *Hum Reprod Update.* 2011;17(5):620–7.
6. McCoy RC. Mosaicism in preimplantation human embryos: When chromosomal abnormalities are the norm. *Trends Genet TIG.* Elsevier, 2017;33(7):448–63.
7. Capalbo A et al. Abnormally fertilized oocytes can result in healthy live births: Improved genetic technologies for preimplantation genetic testing can be used to rescue viable embryos in in vitro fertilization cycles. *Fertil Steril.* 2017;108(6):1007–15.e3.
8. Taylor TH et al. The origin, mechanisms, incidence and clinical consequences of chromosomal mosaicism in humans. *Hum Reprod Update.* 2014;20(4):571–81.
9. Gueye NA et al. Uniparental disomy in the human blastocyst is exceedingly rare. *Fertil Steril.* 2014;101(1):232–6.
10. Munne S et al. Treatment-related chromosome abnormalities in human embryos. *Hum Reprod.* 1997;12(4):780–4.
11. Liu J et al. DNA microarray reveals that high proportions of human blastocysts from women of advanced maternal age are aneuploid and mosaic. *Biol Reprod.* 2012;87(6):148.
12. Nakai-Futatsugi Y, Niwa H. Epiblast and primitive endoderm differentiation: Fragile specification ensures stable commitment. *Cell Stem Cell.* 2015;16(4):346–7.
13. Delhanty JDA et al. Detection of aneuploidy and chromosomal mosaicism in human embryos during preimplantation sex determination by fluorescent *in situ* hybridisation (FISH). *Hum Mol Genet.* 1993;2(8):1183–5.
14. Greco E, Minasi MG, Fiorentino F. Healthy babies after intrauterine transfer of mosaic aneuploid blastocysts. *N Engl J Med.* 2015;373(21):2089–90.
15. Munné S, Grifo J, Wells D. Mosaicism: "survival of the fittest" versus "no embryo left behind". *Fertil Steril.* 2016;105(5):1146–9.
16. Spinella F et al. Extent of chromosomal mosaicism influences the clinical outcome of in vitro fertilization treatments. *Fertil Steril.* 2018;109(1):77–83.
17. Victor AR et al. One hundred mosaic embryos transferred prospectively in a single clinic: Exploring when and why they result in healthy pregnancies. *Fertil Steril.* 2019;111(2):280–93.
18. Goodrich D et al. A randomized and blinded comparison of qPCR and NGS-based detection of aneuploidy in a cell line mixture model of blastocyst biopsy mosaicism. *J Assist Reprod Genet.* 2016;33(11):1473–80.
19. Popovic M et al. Extended *in vitro* culture of human embryos demonstrates the complex nature of diagnosing chromosomal mosaicism from a single trophectoderm biopsy. *Hum Reprod.* 2019;34(4):758–69.
20. Capalbo A et al. Detecting mosaicism in trophectoderm biopsies: Current challenges and future possibilities. *Hum Reprod.* 2016;32(3):492–8.
21. Capalbo A, Rienzi L. Mosaicism between trophectoderm and inner cell mass. *Fertil Steril.* 2017;107(5):1098–106.
22. Weissman A et al. Chromosomal mosaicism detected during preimplantation genetic screening: Results of a worldwide web-based survey. *Fertil Steril.* 2017;107(5):1092–7.

23. Gonzalez-Merino E et al. Incidence of chromosomal mosaicism in human embryos at different developmental stages analyzed by fluorescence in situ hybridization. *Genet Test.* 2003;7(2):85–95.

24. Daphnis DD et al. Detailed FISH analysis of day 5 human embryos reveals the mechanisms leading to mosaic aneuploidy. *Hum Reprod.* 2005;20(1):129–37.

25. Baart EB et al. Preimplantation genetic screening reveals a high incidence of aneuploidy and mosaicism in embryos from young women undergoing IVF. *Hum Reprod.* 2006;21(1):223–33.

26. Santos MA et al. The fate of the mosaic embryo: Chromosomal constitution and development of Day 4, 5 and 8 human embryos. *Hum Reprod.* 2010;25(8):1916–26.

27. Treff NR et al. SNP microarray-based 24 chromosome aneuploidy screening is significantly more consistent than FISH. *Mol Hum Reprod.* May 21, 2010;16(8):583–9.

28. Van der Aa N et al. Genome-wide copy number profiling of single cells in S-phase reveals DNA-replication domains. *Nucleic Acids Res.* 2013;41(6):e66.

29. Huang A et al. Prevalence of chromosomal mosaicism in pregnancies from couples with infertility. *Fertil Steril.* 2009;91(6):2355–60.

30. Jacod BC et al. Does confined placental mosaicism account for adverse perinatal outcomes in IVF pregnancies? *Hum Reprod.* 2008;23(5):1107–12.

31. Barbash-Hazan S et al. Preimplantation aneuploid embryos undergo self-correction in correlation with their developmental potential. *Fertil Steril.* 2009;92(3):890–6.

32. Bazrgar M et al. Self-correction of chromosomal abnormalities in human preimplantation embryos and embryonic stem cells. *Stem Cells Dev.* 2013;22(17):2449–56.

33. Bolton H et al. Mouse model of chromosome mosaicism reveals lineage-specific depletion of aneuploid cells and normal developmental potential. *Nat Commun.* 2016;7:11165.

34. McCoy RC et al. Evidence of selection against complex mitotic-origin aneuploidy during preimplantation development. *PLOS Genet.* 2015;11(10):e1005601.

35. Capalbo A et al. FISH reanalysis of inner cell mass and trophectoderm samples of previously array-CGH screened blastocysts shows high accuracy of diagnosis and no major diagnostic impact of mosaicism at the blastocyst stage. *Hum Reprod.* 2013;28(8):2298–307.

36. Grati FR et al. Chromosomal mosaicism in the fetoplacental unit. *Best Pract Res Clin Obstet Gynaecol.* 2017;42:39–52.

37. Munné S et al. Detailed investigation into the cytogenetic constitution and pregnancy outcome of replacing mosaic blastocysts detected with the use of high-resolution next-generation sequencing. *Fertil Steril.* 2017;108(1):62–71.e8.

38. Fragouli E et al. Analysis of implantation and ongoing pregnancy rates following the transfer of mosaic diploid-aneuploid blastocysts. *Hum Genet.* 2017;136(7):805–19.

39. Mardy A, Wapner RJ. Confined placental mosaicism and its impact on confirmation of NIPT results. *Am J Med Genet C Semin Med Genet.* 2016;172(2):118–22.

40. Van Opstal D, Srebniak MI. Cytogenetic confirmation of a positive NIPT result: Evidence-based choice between chorionic villus sampling and amniocentesis depending on chromosome aberration. *Expert Rev Mol Diagn.* 2016;16(5):513–20.

41. Scott RT et al. Comprehensive chromosome screening is highly predictive of the reproductive potential of human embryos: A prospective, blinded, nonselection study. *Fertil Steril.* 2012;97(4):870–5.

42. Yang Z et al. Selection of single blastocysts for fresh transfer via standard morphology assessment alone and with array CGH for good prognosis IVF patients: Results from a randomized pilot study. *Mol Cytogenet.* 2012;5(1):24.

43. Forman EJ et al. In vitro fertilization with single euploid blastocyst transfer: A randomized controlled trial. *Fertil Steril.* 2013;100(1):100–7.e1.

9

Transfer of Mosaic Embryos

Francesco Fiorentino, Ermanno Greco, Maria Giulia Minasi, and Francesca Spinella

CONTENTS

Origin and Frequency of Chromosomal Mosaicism

Embryonic mosaicism is a phenomenon characterized by the presence of karyotypically different cell lines within the same embryo. It is relatively common in human preimplantation embryos and may occur with regard to numerical aberrations and/or structural aneuploidy [1]. Chromosomal mosaicism may refer to embryos composed with two or more different abnormal cell lines (e.g., mosaic−aneuploid), or with normal and abnormal cell lines (e.g., euploid/aneuploid mosaic) [1,2].

Euploid/aneuploid mosaicism may occur by mitotic errors arising after fertilization of normal gametes. Conversely, it may originate as a meiotic non-disjunction event, leading to a trisomic conceptus, followed be a second post-zygotic event (trisomy rescue) [1,3−9] (Figure 9.1). Mitotic events that lead to mosaicism may include anaphase lag, mitotic nondisjunction, inadvertent chromosome demolition, or premature cell division before DNA duplication [6,10−12]. Some fluorescence in situ hybridization (FISH) studies suggest that mosaic embryos are the result of mitotic non-disjunction, with only 5% being due to other mechanisms, such as anaphase lag [13]. Subsequent studies using whole-genome hybridization and modern sequencing approaches have revealed that most of the diploid−aneuploid embryos are affected by single chromosome gains or losses or both [12,14,15] (Figure 9.2).

Due to the nature of mitotic errors, the distribution and the number of aneuploid cells within the embryos could vary during embryo development. For example, if mitotic errors occur at the time of the first or second cleavage, or if the original error is meiotic in origin, mosaic embryos will be composed of a greater proportion of abnormal cells than errors occurring during the third cleavage [16,17]. Studies examining different sections of the same blastocyst or assessing the chromosomes of single-cell biopsies showed that there is no evidence for a preferential allocation of aneuploid cells to the trophectoderm of mosaic blastocyst-stage human embryos. However, there remains a possibility that random distribution of abnormal cells could, by chance, leave the inner cell mass (ICM) unaffected and be present in trophectoderm (TE) only, or vice-versa [1,18] (Figure 9.3). Recent studies provided evidence that such events may occur when euploid/aneuploidy mosaic embryos are affected by low-level mosaicism [14,19]. In contrast, mosaic embryos with elevated levels of aneuploid cells show higher chances to have chromosome abnormalities distributed in the entirety of the embryo [19,20].

A number of recent studies have investigated the frequency of mosaicism in human preimplantation embryos using FISH and/or contemporary methods for 24-chromosome analysis. These studies indicate that the incidence of mosaic embryos may vary based on the sensitivity of the analysis used, patient

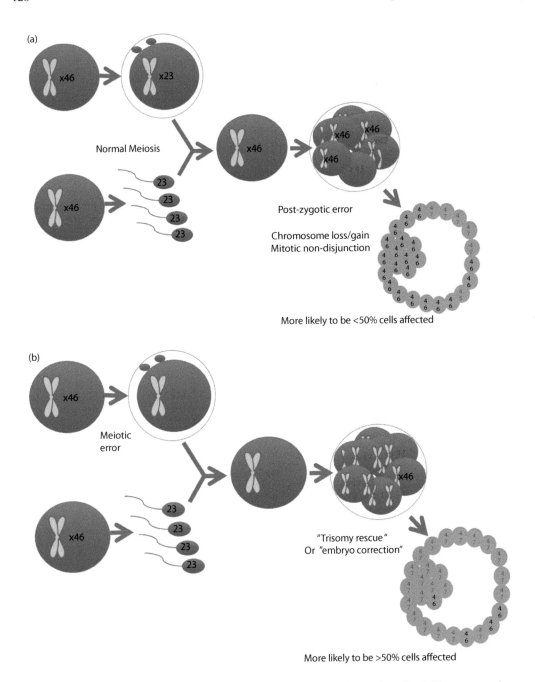

FIGURE 9.1 Origin of mosaicism in preimplantation embryos. (a) Normal fertilization of euploid gametes produces a diploid, chromosomally normal zygote. Errors in mitosis during embryonic cell divisions lead to a mixture of euploid and aneuploid cells. (b) Meiotic errors occurring in gametes (female meiosis-I error or meiosis-II or male meiosis may also occur), resulting in embryos comprised of homogeneously aneuploidy cells (i.e., aneuploid karyotype) followed by a second event of "trisomy rescue" or embryo correction.

cohorts (i.e., the proportion of embryos that are euploid/aneuploid mosaics decreases with increasing maternal age), laboratory conditions, and may depend on the developmental stage of the embryo (cleavage stage or blastocyst stage).

Initial studies to investigate the frequency of embryonic mosaicism were performed by FISH analysis. These studies reported that mosaicism ranged from 18% to 46% at blastocyst stage [2,16,21–24] and

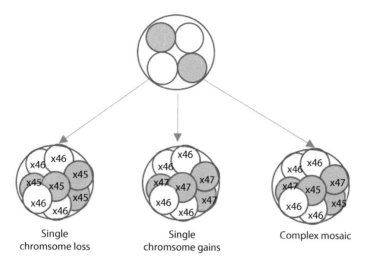

FIGURE 9.2 Composition of diploid–aneuploid mosaic embryos. Aneuploidy in mosaic embryos may be affected by single chromosome copy number losses or single chromosome gains, or complex mosaic aneuploidies when more than one kind of abnormal cell lines coexist with normal cell lines.

from 30% to 90% at cleavage-stage level [5,17]. However, the FISH technique produces a high number of technical artifacts. These technical issues may affect the accuracy of the results and could potentially have introduced an overestimation of the mosaicism rate. Moreover, FISH screens for a minority of chromosomes—those most commonly observed in pregnancy loss and aneuploid deliveries—which are not necessarily the most relevant for early embryos.

The introduction of recent molecular techniques for comprehensive chromosome screening (CCS) in embryos, such as single-nucleotide polymorphism (SNP) arrays, array comparative genome hybridization (aCGH), and next-generation sequencing (NGS), provided more clear information on mosaicism, indicating that the rate of mosaicism is lower than those previously reported by FISH analysis.

Studies assessing cleavage-stage embryos showed that the incidence of diploid–aneuploid mosaic embryos ranges between 15% and 90% [4,6,26] and is lower at blastocyst stage, where the incidence ranges from 3% to 30% [1,9,14,19,27–32] (Table 9.1).

Although meiotic aneuploidy increases with age, there is no clear relationship between maternal age and mosaicism that arises solely by mitotic errors [12,33–35]. It has been hypothesized that advancing female age does not influence the incidence of post-zygotic chromosome abnormalities, although the increasing likelihood of meiotic aneuploidy with increasing maternal age means that the proportion of embryos that are euploid/aneuploid mosaics decreases with age, from 26.6% in women <35 years old to

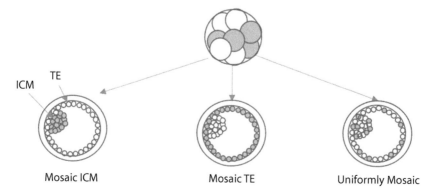

FIGURE 9.3 Theoretical aneuploidy distribution of mosaic blastocyst-stage human embryos. Aneuploid cells could be confined on inner cell mass (ICM) or in trophectoderm (TE), or in both (uniformly mosaic).

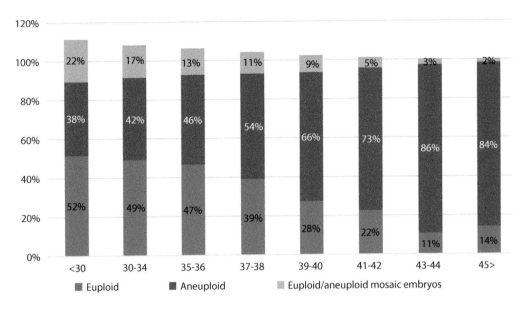

FIGURE 9.4 Distribution of embryos by age group and diagnosis.

TABLE 9.1

Frequency of Euploid/Aneuploidy Mosaic Embryos

Cleavage Stage			Blastocyst Stage			
FISH%	aCGH%	SNP%	FISH%	aCGH%	SNP%	NGS%
15–90	70	31–60	3–17	3–15	4–19	9–30

Abbreviations: aCGH, array comparative genomic hybridization; FISH, fluorescence *in situ* hybridization; NGS, next-generation sequencing; SNP, single-nucleotide polymorphism.

10.5% in >42-year-old women [35]. In agreement with these findings, a recent study demonstrated that a drastic reduction in the proportion of mosaic embryos compared to aneuploid embryos was observed in women with advanced maternal age. This reduction was paralleled by a reduction in the proportion of euploid embryos in the same patient's cohort [36] (Figure 9.4).

Studies on the chromosomal composition of mosaic embryos reported that aneuploidy might affect all chromosomes and involve one or more of them. In addition, a small excess of post-zygotic chromosome gain compared to loss has been reported [1], while this difference was not evident at cleavage-stage embryo [13]. Apart from numerical abnormalities, structural abnormalities may also occur in cleavage-stage human embryos, leading to partial mosaicism of certain chromosomal segments [10,14]. Recent research has given considerable attention to segmental abnormalities. In over 29,000 embryos biopsied using NGS, 7.34% showed mosaic segmental abnormalities [14]. Moreover, in their investigation, Vera-Rodriguez and coauthors revealed that mosaic structural abnormalities are present in 29/84 (34.5%) of the biopsied TE cells [37]. They performed FISH analysis of additional cells from the corresponding embryos and confirmed that cells with segmental chromosome abnormalities and normal cells were present in the same embryos, suggesting that the aneuploidies were likely of mitotic origin [37].

Viability of Mosaic Embryos and Clinical Outcome

Chromosomal mosaicism, similar to a full aneuploid condition, is believed to be directly responsible for the high rates of early human pregnancy failures in both spontaneous conceptions and after *in vitro* fertilization (IVF) treatments. Mosaicism has been suggested to affect the developmental potential of human preimplantation embryos, possibly leading to developmental arrest or implantation failure or result in fetal or confined placental mosaicism [17]. It might also cause congenital malformations, mental retardation, and uniparental disomy [17]. As such, until recently, mosaic embryos obtained after IVF treatment were not considered suitable for transfer.

The introduction of new technologies for preimplantation genetic testing for aneuploidies (PGT-A), combined with trophectoderm biopsy of blastocysts, have improved detection of chromosomal mosaicism, introducing a revolution in our knowledge of mosaic embryo viability. Indeed, applying aCGH- and NGS-based PGT-A, recent studies demonstrated that euploid/diploid mosaic embryos hold the potential to implant and result in the birth of healthy babies [14,30,32,34,38]. Since then, many reproductive genetics laboratories are now routinely including embryonic mosaicism on their diagnostic reports. These findings have generated an extensive debate on mosaic embryos. Criticisms were raised on the utility to detect and report chromosomal mosaicism and whether mosaic embryos should be transferred or not.

The first prospective study providing information on the developmental potential of mosaic diploid–aneuploid blastocysts was carried out by Greco and colleagues (Table 9.2) [30]. In this prospective study, aCGH was used to classify embryos, and 18 euploid/aneuploid mosaic embryos were transferred in those women who did not have any euploid embryos available for transfer. The implantation rate for mosaic embryos was 44% (8/18), and the live birth rate was 33% (6/18). All pregnancies that went to term were confirmed through sampling of the chorionic villi to have a normal karyotype [30].

After the Greco report, several other studies involving the transfer of larger numbers of mosaic embryos have been performed [14,32,38,39]. These studies confirmed that mosaic embryos have some level of developmental competence, and reported similar implantation, miscarriage, and pregnancy rates (Table 9.2). The developmental potential of mosaic embryos was further examined comparing the outcome of mosaic embryos with those of a matched euploid control group. This study demonstrated that mosaic blastocysts have a significantly lower implantation (38.5% vs. 54.6%, p = 0.02), and a lower ongoing pregnancy rate (30% vs. 46.4%, p = 0.014) as compared to euploid embryos [32].

Retrospective studies further confirmed the low reproductive potential of mosaic embryos, reporting a reduced implantation rate, pregnancy rate, and increased miscarriage rates compared to euploid embryos [14,38,39]. These studies [14,32,38,39] investigated the impact of aneuploid/euploid cell ratio on mosaic embryo development. Spinella and coauthors demonstrated that blastocysts with <50% mosaicism show a significant reduction in ongoing pregnancy rate and baby born rate compared to those with >50% mosaicism. Other studies reported that there was a tendency for mosaics with 40%–80% abnormal cells to have a lower ongoing implantation rate than those with <40% (22% vs. 56%) [14–38]. In contrast, a study from Victor et al. reported that the percentage of aneuploid cells in TE biopsies did not correlate with the clinical outcome. Indeed, no significant difference was observed between mosaic embryos with 20%–40% mosaicism and those with 40%–80% mosaicism in terms of implantation and pregnancy rate [39]. Interestingly, a recent comprehensive analysis of mosaic embryo clinical outcomes [40], in which data from more than 300 transfers of mosaic embryos were combined, provided strong evidence that embryos with a low fraction of abnormal cells (<50%) have higher chances of resulting in viable embryos compared to embryos with a high fraction of abnormal cells (>50%).

It is important to note that, due to the intrinsic nature of mosaicism, the chromosomal makeup achieved from a TE biopsy only represents a snapshot of a small portion of the embryo and does not necessarily reflect the karyotype of the entire embryo. In this view, the mosaicism level deduced from

TABLE 9.2

Clinical Outcome after Transfer of Mosaic Embryos

	No. of Mosaic Blastocysts Transferred	No. of Transfers	Implantation Rate (%)	Miscarriage Rate (%)	Pregnancy Rate (%)
Greco et al. [30]	18	18	44	11	33
Fragouli et al. [38]	44	39	30.1	55.6	15.4
Munnè et al. [14]	143	138	53	24	41
Spinella et al. [32]	78	77	38.5	7.8	30
Victor et al. [39]	100	83	38	7	30

a single TE biopsy might not unequivocally represent the exact mosaicism percentage of the remaining TE cells or the inner cell mass constitution. Whether data on mosaicism obtained from a small portion of the embryo may predict the chromosomal status of the remainder of the embryo still remains an important open question. Further studies are welcome to demonstrate the correspondence between mosaicism results obtained from TE biopsies performed in different sides of the embryos and the inner cell mass or the whole embryo.

Concerning the clinical outcome of mosaic embryos with different categories of aneuploidies, studies concordantly reported that there was no difference in the clinical outcome between monosomic and trisomic mosaics, but mosaic blastocysts carrying multiple chromosome abnormalities (complex mosaic) had the lowest viability among the mosaic embryos [32,38]. Recently, in a larger analysis of more than 300 mosaic embryos, it was reported that complex and single segmental mosaics fared better than all other types—namely, those affecting multiple segmental gains/losses—or one or two whole chromosomes [40]. However, follow-up data obtained so far are still not sufficient to draw a definitive conclusion on the influence of different chromosomes in mosaic embryo development.

A still unresolved issue concerns the chance of preimplantation mosaicism to result in congenital abnormalities and the birth of affected children. To date, over 150 pregnancies have been obtained, all with a normal fetal karyotype [14,38,39,40]. Although high, this is still an insufficient number to draw any conclusion. Moreover, to verify the possible impact of mosaicism, there is certainly a need for comprehensive analyses of obstetrical and neonatal outcome and long-term follow-up data of child obtained after transfer of mosaic embryos, should be karyotyped and followed for years through the child's development, examining cells from different tissue. The lack of this information impairs a definitive conclusion on the impact of mosaicism on embryo development. For these reasons, transfers involving mosaic diploid–aneuploid blastocysts should only be undertaken with caution and after appropriate counseling [41,42].

Patients considering transfer of mosaic embryos must receive thorough genetic counseling about potential pregnancy risks and outcomes; they should be made aware that these mosaic embryos may be characterized by decreased implantation and pregnancy potential as well as increased risk of genetic abnormalities and adverse pregnancy outcomes. Pretest counseling should include a discussion about the frequency of mosaic results, the challenges associated with interpretation of the results, the possibility of a false positive diagnosis of embryonic mosaicism, and the limited predictive data available. Genetic counseling should also inform the patient that mosaicism found in a TE biopsy may have clinical implications for the pregnancy and/or may result in live births with mosaic aneuploidies. Confirmation of the fetal karyotype by invasive prenatal diagnosis, preferably amniocentesis, should also be suggested for any ensued pregnancy. Experts in the reproductive field recommended prioritization of euploid embryos over mosaic embryos for transfer and only consider mosaics for replacement when no euploid embryos are available [35].

A position statement on the transfer of mosaic embryos proposed by Preimplantation Genetic Diagnosis International Society (PGDIS) [43], and Controversies in Preconception and Prenatal Genetic Diagnosis (CoGEN) [44] suggest favoring transfer of embryos with lower levels (20%–40%) of mosaic aneuploidy [43,44], while discouraging [44] the transfer of mosaics involving chromosomes compatible with live birth in pure aneuploid form (i.e., trisomies for chromosomes X, Y, 13, 18, 21, and 45,XO), associated with uniparental disomy (UPD; chromosomes 7, 14, 15) or intrauterine growth restriction (chromosome 16).

While the influence of the type and the load of aneuploidy in mosaic development are being established, a preponderance of evidence now shows that the mosaic category of blastocysts contains its own distinct set of clinical outcomes, different from the uniform euploid or aneuploid categories. For this reason, experts in the field suggest classification of mosaic embryos as a distinct category in terms of viability, lying in between euploid and fully abnormal embryos (Figure 9.5). This category of mosaic embryos may be characterized by decreased implantation and pregnancy potential as well as increased risk of genetic abnormalities and adverse pregnancy outcomes.

The clinical application of advanced PGT methodologies is now beginning to yield important information on viability for transfer of mosaic embryos, and it is likely that shortly new and more detailed guidelines will be produced to help clinicians and geneticists to support patients with proper genetic counseling.

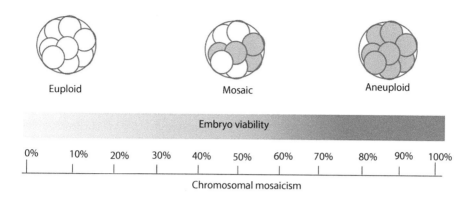

FIGURE 9.5 Viability of mosaic embryos. Mosaic embryos are a category in between euploid and fully chromosomally abnormal embryos in terms of viability. Based on evidence reported by several studies, mosaic viability could be influenced by the percentage of aneuploidy cells within the embryo (i.e., chromosomal mosaicism levels).

Potential Mechanism for Self-Correction of Mosaic Embryos

The concept that a mosaic blastocyst with a high percentage of aneuploid cells is less likely to succeed than one with lower percentage of aneuploid cells was extensively demonstrated in a mouse model [45]. experimental data suggests that aneuploid cells, when present at low levels (<50%), could be progressively depleted from the blastocyst stage onward, leading to the development of normal embryos [45] (Figure 9.6). In this regard, using an extended *in vitro* embryo culture protocol, Papovic et al. investigated the effects of chromosomal aberrations and blastocyst mosaicism on early preimplantation, up to 12 days post-fertilization (dpf). They found that human mosaic blastocysts diagnosed with a high percentage of abnormal cells were more likely to be non-viable at 12 dpf. These findings further support the presence of a mechanism for the depletion of abnormal cells in the embryo outgrowths [46].

Several mechanisms have been proposed to explain the "self-correction" process of mosaic embryos. One of these implicates cell death or reduced proliferation of aneuploid cells compared to euploid cells [47]. Direct evidence revealed by studies in mice showed that depletion of aneuploid blastomeres first becomes apparent during blastocyst maturation, when abnormal ICM cells have increased apoptosis and abnormal TE cells exhibit limited proliferation, prior to implantation and later in the early developing embryo [48]. In Bolton's mouse model, it was shown that the fate of aneuploid cells in early embryos depends on lineage: aneuploid cells in the fetal lineage (i.e., ICM) are eliminated by apoptosis, whereas

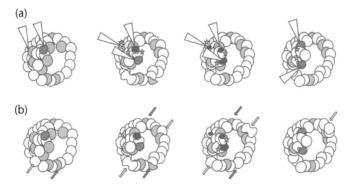

FIGURE 9.6 Elimination of abnormal cells during blastocyst development. Schematic representation of sequential step of chimera (euploid cells in white, aneuploidy cell in blue), representing (a) apoptosis of a aneuploid cells (arrow), followed by engulfment of the apoptotic debris into an efferosome by a neighboring control cell (star); (b) normal cell division of euploid cells (empty arrow) and abnormal cells division of aneuploidy cell (blue arrow).

those in the placental lineage (i.e., TE) showed severe proliferative defects [45] (Figure 9.6). A recent article confirmed that in the human embryo, the dynamics of cell proliferation and death are different, on average, among euploid, mosaic, and aneuploid blastocysts. This could correspond to the proposed self-correction mechanism, as aneuploid cells might proliferate more slowly or undergo apoptosis, and euploid cells compensate by elevating their rates of proliferation [46]. Evidence that could support or refute this notion in human embryos, however, is currently lacking. To date, it is unknown whether minimum threshold proportions of euploid cells are required to support normal development.

The self-correction hypothesis is also supported by the notion that the mosaicism rate is less than 1%–2% in viable pregnancies [49], which suggests that the phenomenon may also occur during intrauterine development to remove abnormal cells from mammalian embryos in the post-implantation period. The mosaic model used by Bolton et al. [45] was generated with a drug introducing massive chromosome abnormalities for multiple chromosome (complex mosaic) and it remains to be determined if mosaicism for one or few chromosomes results in similar effects on cell survival.

Detection of Chromosomal Mosaicism in Human Preimplantation Embryos

The detection of chromosomal mosaicism in preimplantation embryos is technically challenging, and the accuracy of mosaicism predictions is strictly related to the methodology used for genetic testing. The methodology initially applied in preimplantation genetic testing (PGT) for aneuploidy (PGT-A) involved the use of the FISH technique. This approach has several limitations that have hampered accurate detection of aneuploidies. Only in a later stage, CCS methodologies were introduced to overcome FISH limits, including quantitative PCR (qPCR), SNP arrays, aCGH and, most recently, NGS. These advanced PGT assays accurately assess the copy number of all 24 chromosomes from biopsy of a single or multiple cells, delivering results with lower error rates as compared to FISH.

Current PGT-A technologies have the potential to detect chromosomal mosaicism. However, it important to note that this implies the biopsy of multiple cells and is related to the sensitivity of the PGT-A technology. Indeed, given the nature of mosaicism (presence of karyotypically distinct cell lines in the same sample), single-cell biopsy (i.e., single blastomere) from cleavage-stage embryos does not allow the detection of mosaicism. The results of testing in this case will give information only on the blastomere analyzed, which may not be representative of the remainder embryos. In contrast, biopsy at blastocyst stage has the advantage of allowing more cells to be sampled (~5–10 TE cells), making it more likely that the samples biopsied from a mosaic blastocyst include more than one cell line.

Although sampling more embryonic cells, instead of a single blastomere, gives the possibility to detect chromosomal mosaicism occurrences, most methods used for PGT-A lack the sensitivity necessary to detect minor cell populations within the biopsy specimen. The sensitivity of a PGT-A assay is related to its limit of detection (the smallest number of aneuploid cells detectable in a mix of euploid and aneuploid cells) and the software used for the bioinformatic analysis. Methods such as aCGH has been extensively validated for aneuploidy/mosaicism detection. An initial validation study, using known mixtures of euploid and aneuploid (trisomic) cells, demonstrated that aCGH detects mosaic chromosome abnormalities in TE biopsies with relatively high accuracy when the minor cell line represents ~35% or more of the embryonic cells under analysis [50]. In general, TE biopsy specimens in which fewer than 40% of cells have a divergent chromosome number might be incorrectly classified as euploid when using aCGH. These results were also confirmed by reconstruction experiments in which mosaicism was detected at a percentage ranging between 25%–37.5% for gains and 37%–50% for losses [51]. Another study performed by Capalbo et al. [19] demonstrated that aCGH failed to detect diploid–aneuploid mosaicism when <25% of cells in the TE biopsy specimens were abnormal, while it accurately detected all cases of mosaicism when >40% of TE biopsy samples were aneuploid. More recently, Greco et al. demonstrated that aCGH was capable of detecting mosaicism at a 20% level (Table 9.3). Such differences could be related to the quality of DNA obtained from the biopsy. High-quality DNA results in reduced background noise, thus allowing detection of low-level mosaicism [32].

Other PGT methodologies, such as SNP microarray, have also been validated for mosaicism detection. Scott et al. [52] mixed DNA samples extracted from cytogenetically normal and abnormal sources, without whole-genome amplification (WGA), to determine the limits of detection of chromosomal

TABLE 9.3

Limit of Detection of Aneuploidy Cells in Diploid/Aneuploidy Mosaic Embryo

	aCGH%	SNP%	NGS%	qPCR%
Scott et al. [52]		>20–30		
Northrop et al. [29]		>40–60		
Mamas et al. [50]	>25			
Capalbo et al. [19]	>40			
Novik et al. [51]	>25			
Maxwell et al. [59]			>20	
Greco et al. [30]	>20			
Goodrich et al. [60]			>50	>50
Vera-Rodriguez et al. [37]			>11[a]	
Munnè et al. [34]			>20[a]	
Spinella et al. [32]			>20	

Abbreviations: aCGH, array comparative genomic hybridization; SNP, single nucleotide polymorphism; NGS, next generation sequencing; qPCR, quantitative polymerase chain reaction.

[a] Whole and segmental aneuploidies.

mosaicism using a 44-K oligonucleotide array. Mosaicism as low as 10% for both gains and losses of whole chromosomes was detectable when data from dye-reversed replicates were combined, but this detection limit rose to 20%–30% mosaicism in the absence of dye-reversed replicates (Table 9.3). Recent studies provide evidence that NGS-based methods have a substantially increased sensitivity for chromosomal mosaicism and therefore the most powerful ability to identify mosaicism [53,54]. Experimental reconstruction models demonstrated that NGS allows the detection of whole and partial chromosomal mosaicism down to a 20% level [32,37] (Table 9.3).

Due to its increased dynamic range in comparison to aCGH, NGS has a greater ability to detect mosaicism in multicellular samples also in the presence of a low level of mosaicism [53]. This was also demonstrated by a recent study reporting that mosaic embryos with 20%–50% of aneuploidy and several embryos with segmental aneuploidy (≥10 Mbp) were hard to distinguish using the aCGH platform, but could be clearly identified using the NGS platform [55].

The detection of mosaicism within an embryo may be subject to some degree of sampling error, technical errors, and erroneous data interpretation. The presence of this potential error has created criticism of the diagnostic accuracy of mosaicism detection. Opponents to chromosomal mosaicism have concerns about its clinical utility, claiming that false positives may arise because of technical artifacts. These artifacts are expected to be introduced by the WGA technique, used to amplify embryonic DNA as first step of the PGT-A process [56–58], or by PGT-A on low-input DNA samples [58]. In this case, artifacts might be misinterpreted as true mosaic aneuploidy and potentially result in discarding euploid embryos, thus causing a decrease in the cumulative live-birth rate [25].

Although WGA artifacts could potentially occur, the use of properly validated PGT-A platforms capable of analyzing mosaic results has the potential to reduce the risk of misdiagnosis due to technical errors. Validation studies have been performed for aCGH [30,50,51] and more recently for NGS [14,32,37–39], demonstrating that these PGT-A platforms are able to reliably detect mosaicism on embryos with a very low level of false positive or false negative results.

Concluding Remarks

Although the significance of mosaicism at the embryo stage is still unclear, it is reasonable to assume that mosaicism will influence the likelihood of success of IVF treatments. It is important to consider that most of the chromosomal screening currently used may fail to detect mosaicism, classifying embryos as euploid or aneuploid. Undetected mosaicism may result in the transfer of embryos with a lower developmental potential compared to full euploid embryos. In contrast, labeling mosaic embryos as fully aneuploid may result in discarding a normal embryo. The introduction of advanced PGT-A technologies such as NGS allows accurate identification of mosaic embryos, thus substantially reducing the risk of discarding potentially viable embryos. This represents an important achievement, especially for patients with poor ovarian reserve, producing a limited number of embryos, or for those in which only chromosomally abnormal embryos have been detected, that represent the majority of IVF patients. Although further studies are needed to strengthen the preliminary results obtained, the transfer of mosaic embryos may give patients a chance to achieve a viable pregnancy. However, this practice should be used with caution and after a proper genetic counseling session.

Accurate detection of mosaicism among embryos may also reduce the risk of early miscarriages and may increase implantation rates following transfer. To date, several issues, such as how mosaic embryos may "self-correct" and if preimplantation mosaicism may result in the birth of affected children, are still unresolved. More studies are welcome to provide better insights into the developmental genetics of mosaic embryos.

REFERENCES

1. Fragouli E et al. Cytogenetic analysis of human blastocysts with the use of FISH, CGH and aCGH: Scientific data and technical evaluation. *Hum Reprod.* 2011;26:480–90.
2. Delhanty JD et al. Detection of aneuploidy and chromosomal mosaicism in human embryos during preimplantation sex determination by fluorescent *in situ* hybridization (FISH). *Hum Mol Genet.* 1993;2:1183–5.
3. Voullaire L, Slater H, Williamson R, Wilton L. Chromosome analysis of blastomeres from human embryos by using comparative genomic hybridization. *Hum Genet.* 2000;106:210–7.
4. Wells D, Delhanty JD. Comprehensive chromosomal analysis of human preimplantation embryos using whole genome amplification and single cell comparative genomic hybridization. *Mol Hum Reprod.* 2000;6:1055–62.
5. Baart E et al. Preimplantation genetic screening reveals a high incidence of aneuploidy and mosaicism in embryos from young women undergoing IVF. *Hum Reprod.* 2006;21:223–33.
6. Mantzouratou A et al. Variable aneuploidy mechanisms in embryos from couples with poor reproductive histories undergoing preimplantation genetic screening. *Hum Reprod.* 2007;22:1844–53.
7. Vanneste E et al. Chromosome instability is common in human cleavage-stage embryos. *Nat Med.* 2009;15:577–83.
8. Sandalinas M, Sadowy S, Alikani M, Calderon G, Cohen J, Munné S. Developmental ability of chromosomally abnormal human embryos to develop to the blastocyst stage. *Hum Reprod.* 2001;16:1954–8.
9. Fragouli E, Lenzi M, Ross R, Katz-Jaffe M, Schoolcraft WB, Wells D. Comprehensive molecular cytogenetic analysis of the human blastocyst stage. *Hum Reprod.* 2008;23:2596–608.
10. Daphnis DD, Delhanty JD, Jerkovic S, Geyer J, Craft I, Harper JC. Detailed FISH analysis of day 5 human embryos reveals the mechanisms leading to mosaic aneuploidy. *Hum Reprod.* 2005;20:129–37.
11. Mantikou E, Wong KM, Repping S, Mastenbroek S. Molecular origin of mitotic aneuploidies in preimplantation embryos. *Biochim Biophys Acta.* 2012;1822:1921–30.
12. van Echten-Arends J et al. Chromosomal mosaicism in human preimplantation embryos: A systematic review. *Hum Reprod Update.* 2011;17:620–7.
13. Munné S. Preimplantation genetic diagnosis of numerical and structural chromosome abnormalities. *Reprod Biomed Online.* 2002;4:183–96.
14. Munne, S et al. Detailed investigation into the cytogenetic constitution and pregnancy outcome of replacing mosaic blastocysts detected with the use of high-resolution next-generation sequencing. *Fertil Steril.* 2017;108:62–71.
15. Vera-Rodriguez M, Rubio C. Assessing the true incidence of mosaicism in preimplantation embryos. *Fertil Steril.* 2017;107:1107–12.
16. Munne S, Weier HU, Grifo J, Cohen J. Chromosome mosaicism in human embryos. *Biol Reprod.* 1994;51:373–9.

17. Taylor TH, Gitlin SA, Patrick JL, Crain JL, Wilson JM, Griffin DK. The origin, mechanisms, incidence and clinical consequences of chromosomal mosaicism in humans. *Hum Reprod Update*. 2014;20:571–81.

18. Fragouli E, Munne S, Wells D. The cytogenetic constitution of human blastocysts: Insights from comprehensive chromosome screening strategies. *Hum Reprod Update*. 2019;25:15–33.

19. Capalbo A, Wright G, Elliott T, Ubaldi FM, Rienzi L, Nagy ZP. FISH reanalysis of inner cell mass and trophectoderm samples of previously array-CGH screened blastocysts shows high accuracy of diagnosis and no major diagnostic impact of mosaicism at the blastocyst stage. *Hum Reprod*. 2013;28: 2298–307.

20. Capalbo A, Rienzi L. Mosaicism between trophectoderm and inner cell mass. *Fertil Steril*. 2017;107:1098–106.

21. Magli MC, Jones GM, Gras L, Gianaroli L, Korman I, Trouson AO. Chromosome mosaicism in day 3 aneuploid embryos that develop to morphologically normal blastocysts *in vitro*. *Hum Reprod*. 2000;15:1781–6.

22. Bielanska M, Tan SL, Ao A. Chromosomal mosaicism throughout human Preimplantation development in vitro: Incidence, type, and relevance to embryo outcome. *Hum Reprod*. 2002;17:413–9.

23. Munne S. Chromosome abnormalities and their relationship to morphology and development of human embryos. *Reprod Biomed Online*. 2006;12:234–53.

24. Colls P, Escudero T, Cekleniak N, Sadowy S, Cohen J, Munne S. Increased efficiency of preimplantation genetic diagnosis for infertility using "no result rescue". *Fertil Steril*. 2007;88:53–61.

25. Gleicher N et al. Accuracy of preimplantation genetic screening (PGS) is compromised by degree of mosaicism of human embryos. International PGS Consortium Study Group. *Reprod Biol Endocrinol*. 2016;14:54.

26. Treff NR, Su J, Tao X, Levy B, Scott RT Jr. Accurate single cell 24 chromosome aneuploidy screening using whole genome amplification and single nucleotide polymorphism microarrays. *Fertil Steril*. 2010;94:2017–21.

27. Johnson DS et al. Preclinical validation of a microarray method for full molecular karyotyping of blastomeres in a 24-h protocol. *Hum Reprod*. 2010;25:1066–75.

28. Johnson DS et al. Comprehensive analysis of karyotypic mosaicism between trophectoderm and inner cell mass. *Mol Hum Reprod*. 2010;169:44–949.

29. Northrop LE, Treff NR, Levy B, Scott Jr RT. SNP microarray-based 24 chromosome aneuploidy screening demonstrates that cleavage-stage FISH poorly predicts aneuploidy in embryos that develop to morphologically normal blastocysts. *Mol Hum Reprod*. 2010;16:590–600.

30. Greco E, Minasi MG, Fiorentino F. Healthy babies born after intrauterine transfer of mosaic aneuploid blastocyst. *NEJM*. 2015;373:2089–90.

31. Ruttanajit T et al. Detection and quantitation of chromosomal mosaicism in human blastocysts using copy number variation sequencing. *Prenat Diagn*. 2016;36:154–62.

32. Spinella F et al. The extent of chromosomal mosaicism influences the clinical outcome of in vitro fertilization treatments. *Fertil Steril*. 2018;109:77–83.

33. Mertzanidou A et al. Microarray analysis reveals abnormal chromosomal complements in over 70% of 14 normally developing human embryos. *Hum Reprod*. 2013;28:256–64.

34. Munné S, Wells D. Detection of mosaicism at blastocyst stage with the use of high-resolution next-generation sequencing. *Fertil Steril*. 2017;107:1085–91.

35. Munné S, Grifo J, Wells D. Mosaicism: "Survival of the fittest" versus "no embryo left behind". *Fertil Steril*. 2016;105:1146–9.

36. Fiorentino F. Biological origin and clinical relevance of the mosaic embryo: origin and fate of aneuploid cells. ESHRE Campus 2019 Athens.

37. Vera-Rodriguez M et al. Distribution patterns of segmental aneuploidies in human blastocysts identified by next-generation sequencing. *Fertil Steril*. 2016;105:1047–55.

38. Fragouli E et al. Analysis of implantation and ongoing pregnancy rates following the transfer of mosaic diploid-aneuploid blastocysts. *Hum Genet*. 2017;108:62–71.

39. Victor AR et al. One hundred mosaic embryos transferred prospectively in a single clinic: Exploring when and why they result in healthy pregnancies. *Fertil Steril*. 2019;111:280–93.

40. Viotti M. Mosaic embryos — A comprehensive and powered analysis of clinical outcomes. *ASRM 2019*, Philadelphia.

41. Besser AG, Mounts EL. Counselling considerations for chromosomal mosaicism detected by preimplantation genetic screening. *Reprod Biomed Online.* 2017;34:369–74.

42. Sachdev NM, Maxwell SM, Besser AG, Grifo JA. Diagnosis and clinical management of embryonic mosaicism. *Fertil Steril.* 2017;107:6–11.

43. Cram DS et al. PGDIS position statement on the transfer of mosaic embryos 2019. *Reprod Biomed Online.* 2019;39(Suppl 1):e1–4

44. CoGEN. 2017. COGEN position statement on chromosomal mosaicism detected in preimplantation blastocyst biopsies. https://www.ivfworldwide.com/index.php?option=com_content&view=article& id=733&Itemid=464. (Accessed 20 April 2018).

45. Bolton H et al. Mouse model of chromosome mosaicism reveals lineage-specific depletion of aneuploid cells and normal developmental potential. *Nat Commun.* 2016;7:11165.

46. Popovic M et al. Extended in vitro culture of human embryos demonstrates the complex nature of diagnosing chromosomal mosaicism from a single trophectoderm biopsy. *Hum Reprod.* 2019;34:758–69.

47. Santos MA et al. The fate of the mosaic embryo: Chromosomal constitution and development of Day 4, 5 and 8 human embryos. *Hum Reprod.* 2010;25:1916–26.

48. Lightfoot DA, Kouznetsova A, Mahdy E, Wilbertz J, Höög C. The fate of mosaic aneuploid embryos during mouse development. *Dev Biol.* 2006;289:384–94.

49. Ledbetter DH et al. Cytogenetic results from the US collaborative study on CVS. *Prenat Diagn.* 1992:12:317–45.

50. Mamas T, Gordon A, Brown A, Harper J, Sengupta S. Detection of aneuploidy by array comparative genomic hybridization using cell lines to mimic a mosaic trophectoderm biopsy. *Fertil Steril.* 2012;97:943–7.

51. Novik V et al. The accuracy of chromosomal microarray testing for identification of embryonic mosaicism in human blastocysts. *Mol Cytogenet.* 2014;7:18.

52. Scott SA, Cohen N, Brandt T, Toruner G, Desnick RJ, Edelmann L. Detection of low-level mosaicism and placental mosaicism by oligonucleotide array comparative genomic hybridization. *Genet Med.* 2010;12:85–92.

53. Fiorentino F et al. Application of next-generation sequencing technology for comprehensive aneuploidy screening of blastocysts in clinical preimplantation genetic screening cycles. *Hum Reprod.* 2014;29:2802–13.

54. Fiorentino F et al. Development and validation of a next generation sequencing (NGS)-based protocol for 24-chromosome aneuploidy screening of embryos. *Fertil Steril.* 2014;101:1375–82.

55. Lai HH et al. Identification of mosaic and segmental aneuploidies by next-generation sequencing in preimplantation genetic screening can improve clinical outcomes compared to array-comparative genomic hybridization. *Mol Cytogenet.* 2017; 26;10:14.

56. Esfandiari N, Bunnell ME, Casper RF. Human embryo mosaicism: Did we drop the ball on chromosomal testing? *J Assist Reprod Genet.* 2016;33:1439–44.

57. Treff NR, Franasiak JM. Detection of segmental aneuploidy and mosaicism in the human preimplantation embryo: Technical considerations and limitations. *Fertil Steril.* 2017;107:27–31.

58. Capalbo A, Ubaldi FM, Rienzi L, Scott R, Treff N. Detecting mosaicism in trophectoderm biopsies: Current challenges and future possibilities. *Hum Reprod.* 2017;32:492–8.

59. Maxwell SM, Colls P, Hodes-Wertz B, McCulloh DH, McCaffrey C, Wells D, Munné S, Grifo JA. Why do euploid embryos miscarry? A case-control study comparing the rate of aneuploidy within presumed euploid embryos that resulted in miscarriage or live birth using next-generation sequencing. *Fertil Steril.* 2016;106:1414-9.e5.

60. Goodrich D, Xing T, Tao X, Lonczak A, Zhan Y, Landis J, Zimmerman R, Scott RTJr, Treff NR. Evaluation of comprehensive chromosome screening platforms for the detection of mosaic segmental aneuploidy. *J Assist Reprod Genet.* 2017;34:975-81.

10

Noninvasive Methods of Preimplantation Genetic Testing for Aneuploidies

Luis Navarro-Sánchez, Carmen María García-Pascual, Lucía Martínez-Merino, Carlos Simón, and Carmen Rubio

CONTENTS

Introduction

The most common genetic abnormality in human embryos is aneuploidy. Its incidence ranges from 20% to 80% [1–3], which is much higher than the frequency in any other species. This abnormality is particularly common among embryos produced by *in vitro* fertilization (IVF), from which more than half are aneuploid.

In conventional IVF, selection of the embryo to transfer is based on morphology, generally according to guidelines established by Gardner and Schoolcraft [4]. However, there is weak association between morphology and ploidy status of the embryo [5,6]. Aneuploid embryos can reach the blastocyst stage with optimal morphological scores and thus can be transferred to the maternal uterus. Depending on the type of aneuploidy, some embryos will not implant, others will implant but will end in miscarriage, and a few can result in an affected newborn [7,8]. Thus, aneuploid embryos must be deselected before transfer.

Morphokinetics—time-lapse monitoring of the embryo 24 hours per day in stable conditions—has been also incorporated in IVF to select the best candidate for transfer. Yet, the many published studies on morphokinetics are heterogeneous in design, type of patients, sample size, day of embryo biopsy (and thus morphokinetic parameters evaluated), statistical approach, and outcome measures. While some differences are described in the morphokinetic pattern between euploid and aneuploid embryos, the clinical significance of these results is absent to modest. No single or combined morphokinetic parameter has been consistently identified as predictive of embryo ploidy status with sufficient sensitivity and/or specificity for clinical embryo selection. Therefore, this system does not allow prediction of the ploidy status of embryos [9].

Hence molecular analysis of embryo chromosomal status remains the best option to select candidates for transfer. This approach distinguishes between euploid embryos, which have the highest implantation potential and ongoing pregnancy rates, and aneuploid embryos, which must be avoided.

Types of Biopsies

Despite controversy about its limitations, preimplantation genetic testing for aneuploidy (PGT-A) is currently the most reliable method to assess chromosomal status of preimplantation embryos. PGT-A can be applied to different preimplantation developmental stages, including the first and second polar bodies (PBs), blastomeres from cleavage-stage embryos on day 3 (D3), and trophectoderm (TE) biopsies. Each stage has specific diagnostic advantages as well as critical limitations that relate to aneuploidy genesis during both meiosis and the preimplantation period of embryo development.

- *PB biopsy:* Removal of the first and/or second PB is an indirect strategy to infer genetic or chromosomal status of the oocyte since only maternal mutations are evaluated. Both PBs are not required for successful fertilization or normal embryonic development. PB biopsy can be an option to avoid ethical restrictions in some countries where embryo genetic analysis is not allowed [10]. However, this strategy fails to capture as many as one in three embryonic aneuploidies [11].
- *Blastomere biopsy:* This approach allows identification of both maternal and paternal contributions. Cleavage-stage biopsy involves removal of a single blastomere from a D3 embryo, usually with six to eight cells and a low fragmentation degree (<20%). For a successful blastomere biopsy, the cell removed from the embryo should be intact and contain a single, visible nucleus. In addition, further development of the embryo should not be impaired because of the biopsy procedure [12], allowing transfer 2 days later, on D5. The main point of discussion on performing genetic analysis on D3 is whether one cell is representative of the entire embryo due to possible mosaicism (i.e., presence of two or more chromosomally distinct cell lines) and the impact on embryo viability and implantation potential [13].
- *Blastocyst biopsy:* This approach also allows identification of both maternal and paternal contributions. It offers the advantage of removing several cells (4–10 cells) from the TE for analysis without affecting the inner cell mass, which will later form the fetus. This avoids risk of affecting fetal development. Analysis of more cells increases the probability to detect mosaicism in the embryo. This upgraded form of PGT-A significantly improves implantation, both with fresh transfer or after vitrification [14,15].
- *Blastocentesis:* This new type of biopsy is thought to be less invasive because it is based on analysis of aspirated blastocoel fluid (BF; i.e., fluid contained in the blastocyst cavity) [16]. Therefore, no cells from the embryo are retrieved. Nevertheless, blastocentesis is an invasive procedure that requires embryo manipulation at the expanded blastocyst stage. The retrieved volume is low (less than 1 µL), and DNA quantity and integrity in the BF remain unknown. Different studies have analyzed BF and TE (currently the gold-standard) for the same embryo and compared PGT-A results from both sources, showing highly variable DNA amplification (34.8% vs. 81.9%, respectively) and concordance rates (37.5% vs. 97.4%, respectively) [17–20]. Consequently, this technique needs further validation to be considered as an alternative to TE biopsy.

All four biopsy approaches require embryo manipulation—the zona pellucida must be perforated in all cases, usually by laser, to retrieve cells or fluids from the embryo. Therefore, specialized equipment, expertly trained operators, and standard protocols are needed to maintain embryo viability [3,21].

Biopsy entails both technical and economic challenges. The high degree of technical skill required to obtain these samples and the cost associated with both equipment and operator training remain a bottleneck for wider implementation of this strategy. In addition, the possibility of harming the embryo is a constant concern for doctors and patients.

Some groups recently proposed a noninvasive approach for PGT-A (niPGT-A) using spent blastocyst medium (SBM) in which the embryo is cultured. This medium, which is discarded in daily routine, contains embryonic cell-free DNA (cfDNA) released by the embryo during the latest stages of preimplantation development. Therefore, it can be used for analysis of its chromosomal content [22].

niPGT-A approaches have various advantages over current strategies, including eliminating costly micromanipulation biopsy procedures and avoiding potential embryo harm associated with cell or fluid removal. Further, niPGT-A would extend the feasibility of PGT-A in many clinics and increase accessibility to a wider population of patients by minimizing laboratory and personnel expenses.

PGT-A Indications

niPGT-A technology could be applied to current indications of PGT-A with high aneuploidy risk, in addition to any IVF patient who wants to increase pregnancy rate and decrease the chance of miscarriage. Current indications of PGT-A include the following.

Advanced Maternal Age

Advanced maternal age (AMA) is the most common indication for PGT-A. Most clinical IVF groups have traditionally considered AMA to be any patient older than 37 years, although recently there is a move to lower the cutoff to 35 years.

Maternal age is a major factor in the prevalence of aneuploidy. The rate of mis-segregation for most clinically relevant aneuploidies (chromosomes 13, 16, and 18) increases from 20% to 60% in women between 35 and 43 years of age [23].

A systematic review and meta-analysis of five randomized controlled trials indicated that PGT-A offered no benefit to AMA patients [24]. However, two prospective randomized trials that evaluated the usefulness of PGT-A in AMA patients showed a significant increase in live birth rates [25,26]. Without aneuploidy screening, AMA patients with a high percentage of aneuploid embryos may be subjected to months of multiple unsuccessful embryo transfers, some of which may end in distressing miscarriages with associated medical risks or in live birth of a child with a chromosomal abnormality [27].

Repetitive Implantation Failure

Repetitive implantation failure (RIF) is defined as three or more failed IVF attempts or failed IVF treatments after cumulative transfer of >10 good-quality embryos. RIF-defining criteria are not homogenous, and an exhaustive and comprehensive definition has not yet been reached. Therefore, RIF remains a challenge to clinicians because it can have multiple causes that are still poorly defined. Further, embryo and endometrial factors can play important roles in this condition. For this indication, despite age, other combined factors can predict higher aneuploidy risk, such as low sperm concentration and low ovarian response [28].

Recurrent Miscarriage

The definition of recurrent miscarriage (RM) varies by country but is generally considered as two to three consecutive miscarriages with a gestational age up to 14 weeks. For PGT-A, other causes of miscarriage should first be discarded with a proper infertility workup, although there is increasing evidence supporting the use of PGT-A. RM couples have an increased number of chromosomally abnormal embryos. Therefore, PGT-A should be recommended when RM is associated with a previous chromosomopathy [29,30].

Severe Male Factor Infertility

Oligozoospermia as well as extreme teratozoospermia are related to increased sperm aneuploidies [31,32]. Testicular sperm from nonobstructive azoospermia and from carriers of Y-chromosome microdeletions also show increased sperm aneuploidy, mostly for sex chromosomes [33,34]. Different types of sperm chromosomal aneuploidies are translated in embryos, and such conditions might partly explain low implantation and high abortion rates observed in these patients [35]. These results highlight severe male factor infertility as a possible referral category for PGT-A.

Previous Trisomic Pregnancy

Some studies suggest that a previous trisomic pregnancy (PTP), whether or not it was viable, is associated with increased risk of another aneuploid conception [36,37]. In particular, individuals <35 years old at the time of the previous pregnancy appear to have an increased risk of future trisomic pregnancies.

Good-Prognosis Patients and Single-Embryo Transfer

For patients with a good prognosis, TE biopsy-based PGT-A could have high potential to increase overall pregnancy rates in IVF programs and to decrease multiple pregnancies when single-embryo transfer (SET) is performed. Three randomized controlled trials comparing blastocyst-stage SET with and without PGT-A in good-prognosis patients showed better clinical pregnancy rates in the PGT-A group and lower miscarriage rates [38–40]. In this group, niPGT-A—which avoids biopsy and thus the derived potential risks for the embryo—could be especially beneficial in combination with SET, as good-prognosis patients present the lowest aneuploidy risk.

Evolution of the Technology

Several methods have been used to study aneuploidies in human embryos. The evolution of aneuploidy screening techniques has provided more reliable and faster results, which enable transfer of euploid embryos even during the same cycle.

From the 1990s to 2010, fluorescence *in situ* hybridization (FISH) was performed on PBs or cleavage-stage embryos. It provided limited information for a few chromosomes [41]. Subsequently, new technologies such as quantitative polymerase chain reaction (qPCR) [42], single-nucleotide polymorphism (SNP) arrays [43], and array comparative genome hybridization (aCGH) [2] facilitated transition to analysis of all 23 chromosome pairs simultaneously in a single cell.

Most recently, decreased cost of genome sequencing has positioned next-generation sequencing (NGS), which also analyzes all 23 chromosome pairs, as the most common technique to study not only aneuploidies but also mitochondrial DNA or gene disorders in simultaneous analyses [44].

NGS starts with whole-genome amplification, followed by a barcoding procedure in which each sample is labeled with unique sequences that permit mixing while allowing samples to be matched to their original source. This barcoding process allows 24–96 samples to be pooled in a sequencing run depending on the platform, optimizing cost per sequenced embryo. Each sequence is aligned with a reference human genome and copy number variations for whole chromosomes, and small deletions/duplications (del/dup) up to 10 Mb are established using specific software. However, NGS cannot detect structural rearrangements in which there is a balanced amount of genetic material, uniparental disomy (both copies of chromosomes are inherited from a single parent), defects affecting the complete set of chromosomes (haploidy, triploidy), and single-gene mutations that cause diseases such as cystic fibrosis.

Today, DNA isolated and amplified from TE and analyzed by NGS is the state of the art of PGT-A [45–49]. In addition, SBM analyzed by NGS is the most common niPGT-A approach.

Analysis of Embryonic Cell-Free DNA in Spent Blastocyst Medium

Shamonki et al. [50] conducted a proof-of-concept study to determine whether cfDNA released by the embryo to the SBM could be used for niPGT-A. For the first time, the authors demonstrated that SBM could render similar results to TE biopsy, although the number of successful concordant samples was low.

Other groups have followed the same strategy of comparing niPGT-A results from SBM and usually TE from the same embryo, with various results (Table 10.1).

TABLE 10.1

Methodological Details of Published niPGT-A Studies Comparing PGT-A Results from SBM and TE Biopsy[a] for the same Embryo

Reference	Number of Samples	Amplification Rate	Concordance Rate	Discordances	Volume of Culture Drop (μL)	Embryo Manipulation	Time in Culture	WGA Method	PGT-A Technique
Shamonki et al. [50]	57	96.5 (55/57)	33.3 (2/6)[b]	—	15	Assisted hatching on D3	D3 to D5/6	Repli-G single cell kit (Qiagen)	aCGH
Xu et al. [51]	42	100 (42/42)	85.7 (36/42)	4 false positives, 2 false negatives	30 (5–20 analysed)	Vitrified on D3	D3 to D5	MALBAC (Yikon)	NGS
Feichtinger et al. [52]	22	81.8 (18/22)	72.2 (13/18)	1 false positive, 4 false negatives	25 (5 analysed)	Assisted hatching on D3	D1 to D5/6	SurePlex (Illumina)	aCGH
Vera-Rodríguez et al. [53]	56	91.1 (51/56)	33.3 (17/51)	—	20	Assisted hatching on D3	D3 to D5	SurePlex + ReproSeq (Illumina + Life Technologies)	NGS
Ho et al. [54]	40	92.5 (37/40)	65.0 (26/40)	8 false positives, 3 false negatives	25 (5 analysed)	Pilot arm: assisted hatching on D3 + cryopreservation Clinical arm: no handling, fresh embryos	D1 to D5	PicoPlex (Rubicon)	NGS
Rubio et al. [55]	115	93.9 (108/115)	Overall: 78.7 (85/108) D5: 63.0 (17/27) D6/7: 84.0 (68/81)	8 false positives, 1 false negative	10	None	D4 to D5/6/7	ReproSeq (Life Technologies)	NGS

[a] Xu et al. [51] compared whole blastocyst, not TE biopsies. Feichtinger et al. [52] compared PB, not TE biopsies.

[b] Only 6 samples of the 55 that amplified were considered for aCGH. They had the highest DNA concentration. From those, only 2 gave informative results and were concordant, one of them after a reamplification.

- Xu et al. [51] compared SBM and whole blastocyst and obtained good amplification and concordance rates (100% and 85.7%, respectively).
- Feichtinger et al. [52] compared SBM and PB in a small number of samples and found lower rates for amplification and concordance (81.8% and 72.2%, respectively). PBs can only diagnose maternally-derived meiotic aneuploidies, however, and do not detect mitotic aneuploidies, mosaicism, and paternally-derived aneuploidies, which are thought to contribute to 3%–4% of chromosomal aberrations.
- Vera-Rodríguez et al. [53] found good amplification rates (91.1%) but only 33.3% concordance. The authors pointed out that maternal contamination was an important factor to work on to improve this approach.
- Ho et al. [54] also examined whether factors such as assisted hatching and embryo morphology would interfere in this approach. The study included a pilot phase involving analysis of SBM and previously cryopreserved research embryos, and a clinical phase involving patient sample analysis. Assisted hatching and embryo morphology did not seem to have a significant influence on cfDNA concentration in the SBM, and consequently does not appear to be necessary or helpful for detection and sequencing of cfDNA for PGT-A.
- Rubio et al. [55] followed a purely noninvasive approach in which embryos were not previously subjected to assisted hatching, blastocentesis, or any vitrification or biopsy procedure, and thus had an intact zona pellucida. The authors showed very high amplification rates (93.9%) and concordance rates, especially when culturing blastocysts for at least 48 hours (84.0%).

Discrepancies in reported results could be related to different methodologies regarding embryo culture (drop volume and time in culture), blastocyst manipulation (assisted hatching, vitrification), and DNA analysis (amplification and detection methods), as well as different criteria used to define concordance rates. A summary of the design of the concordance studies published is shown in Figure 10.1.

How the embryo is handled is extremely important because it can determine not only the quantity and quality of DNA in the spent culture medium, but also the presence of residual cumulus cells not completely stripped from the oocyte that could lead to contamination with maternal DNA, resulting in false negatives. Feichtinger et al., Vera-Rodríguez et al., and Ho et al. [52–54] observed a large number of these cases. Figure 10.2 represents some examples of NGS in TE and SBM, with different types of concordances.

Nevertheless, other sources of DNA contamination need to be considered—external DNA contamination resulting from plasticware, media, or IVF manipulation is crucial, and caution should be taken to prevent it. Hammond et al. [56] found a consistently low level of DNA contamination (mitochondrial and nuclear) in media controls that had not been exposed to embryos. The authors postulated that the origin of this DNA was contamination during production or caused by protein supplementation, which has high DNA binding affinity. In addition, the presence of residual PBs is a potential source of discrepancies related to gender or complementary aneuploidies [53]. Interestingly, this phenomenon is minimized with delayed placement of embryos in the final culture drop [57].

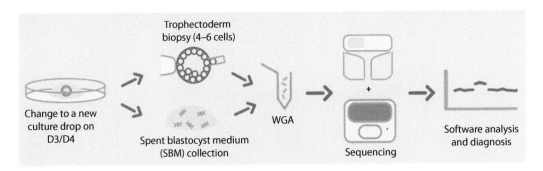

FIGURE 10.1   Workflow of concordance studies between trophectoderm biopsies and spent blastocyst medium (SBM).

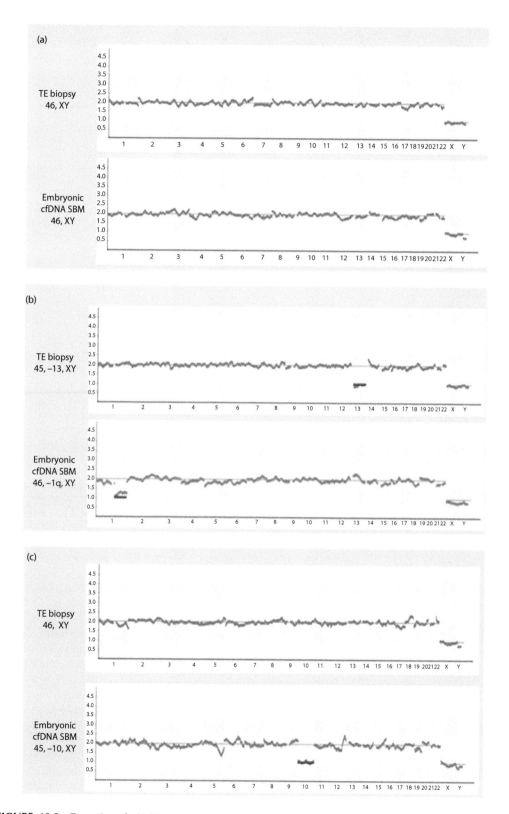

FIGURE 10.2 Examples of niPGT-A results: (a) total concordance; (b) partial concordance; (c) false positive

(Continued)

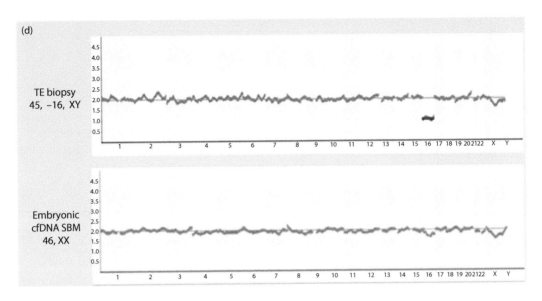

FIGURE 10.2 (CONTINUED)   Examples of niPGT-A results: (d) false negative.

Further, two other studies used a "mixed" approach: for the same embryo, niPGT-A results from BF plus SBM were compared to PGT-A results from TE and whole blastocyst. Kuznyetsov et al. and Li et al. [58,59] obtained high amplification rates (100% and 97.5%, respectively). However, concordance rates differed between BF + SBM and TE (93.0 vs. 45.0%, respectively). In addition, when comparing BF + SBM to whole blastocyst, Kuznyetsov et al. [58] observed an even higher concordance rate (96.4%, although results were not available for all samples), whereas Li et al. [59] reported a much lower rate (50.0%). Therefore, whether BF and SBM could be more representative of the "true" chromosomal content of embryos than TE needs further validation.

Origin of Embryonic Cell-Free DNA in Spent Blastocyst Medium

The origin of embryonic cfDNA remains unclear—we do not know if it comes preferentially from the inner cell mass or TE [58,59]. Further, examining mechanisms implicated in the secretion of cfDNA to media is challenging.

Apoptosis during preimplantation development has been proposed as one potential mechanism since the embryo undergoes rapid dynamic transformation mostly during late preimplantation development that results in high gain and loss of cells, even in genetically healthy embryos [60]. A recent study focused on characterization of DNA retrieved from the BF of expanded blastocysts that had already been diagnosed by TE chromosome analysis and showed higher amplification failure in TE-euploid blastocysts than TE-aneuploid blastocysts, suggesting that higher presence of cfDNA in the internal cavity of TE-aneuploid blastocysts could be related to increased apoptosis [61].

However, our previous publication analyzing embryonic cfDNA released to culture media showed that the amount of cfDNA was not significantly greater in media from aneuploid versus euploid embryos, ruling out this hypothesis. Further, 35% of non-contaminated samples had complementary aneuploidy, suggesting an origin in the PB or mosaicism [53].

DNA also can be successfully amplified in good- and bad-quality embryos, suggesting that expelled cfDNA might reflect general embryo ploidy status in most cases [52]. In that study, in two-thirds of embryos with meiotic aneuploidies detected by PB analysis, at least one chromosomal aberration diagnosed could be detected in the culture medium, making it unlikely that embryonic cells in the culture medium consist solely of extruded aneuploid cells not fully representative of the mosaic embryo.

The results of these two studies contrast with previously published research in mouse embryos showing that mosaic embryos possess certain self-correcting mechanisms to eliminate aneuploid cells through apoptosis during blastocyst development [62].

In conclusion, additional research is needed to understand the mechanisms involved in release of cfDNA to spent culture media. This cfDNA could be as representative of the embryo's chromosomal status as fetal cfDNA circulating in the blood of pregnant women, with high positive predictive value for patients with high aneuploidy risk [63] as well as for the general population [64].

REFERENCES

1. Franasiak JM et al. Aneuploidy across individual chromosomes at the embryonic level in trophectoderm biopsies: Changes with patient age and chromosome structure. *J Assist Reprod Genet.* 2014;31(11):1501–9.
2. Rodrigo L et al. New tools for embryo selection: Comprehensive chromosome screening by array comparative genomic hybridization. *Biomed Res Int.* 2014;2014:517125.
3. Capalbo A et al. Consistent and reproducible outcomes of blastocyst biopsy and aneuploidy screening across different biopsy practitioners: A multicentre study involving 2586 embryo biopsies. *Hum Reprod.* 2016;31(1):199–208.
4. Gardner DK, Schoolcraft WB. In-vitro culture of human blastocyst. In: Jansen R, Mortimer D, eds. *Towards Reproductive Certainty: Fertility and Genetics Beyond.* Carnforth: Parthenon Publishing; 1999:378–88.
5. Alfarawati S et al. The relationship between blastocyst morphology, chromosomal abnormality, and embryo gender. *Fertil Steril.* 2011;95(2):520–4.
6. Capalbo A et al. Correlation between standard blastocyst morphology, euploidy and implantation: An observational study in two centers involving 956 screened blastocysts. *Hum Reprod.* 2014;29(6):1173–81.
7. Rubio C, Pehlivan T, Rodrigo L, Simón C, Remohí J, Pellicer A. Embryo aneuploidy screening for unexplained recurrent miscarriage: A minireview. *Am J Reprod Immunol.* 2005; 53(4):159–65.
8. Campos-Galindo I, García-Herrero S, Martínez-Conejero JA, Ferro J, Simón C, Rubio C. Molecular analysis of products of conception obtained by hysteroembryoscopy from infertile couples. *J Assist Reprod Genet.* 2015;32(5):839–48.
9. Reignier A, Lammers J, Barriere P, Freour T. Can time-lapse parameters predict embryo ploidy? A systematic review. *Reprod Biomed Online.* 2018;36(4):380–7.
10. Geraedts J et al. What next for preimplantation genetic screening? A polar body approach! *Hum Reprod.* 2010;25(3):575–7.
11. Montag M, Köster M, Strowitzki T, Toth B. Polar body biopsy. *Fert Steril.* 2013;100(3):603–7.
12. De Vos A, Van Steirteghem A. Aspects of biopsy procedures prior to preimplantation genetic diagnosis. *Prenat Diagn.* 2001;21(9):767–80.
13. Scott RT Jr, Upham KM, Forman EJ, Zhao T, Treff NR. Cleavage-stage biopsy significantly impairs human embryonic implantation potential while blastocyst biopsy does not: A randomized and paired clinical trial. *Fertil Steril.* 2013;100(3):624–30.
14. Scott KL, Hong KH, Scott RT Jr. Selecting the optimal time to perform biopsy for preimplantation genetic testing. *Fertil Steril.* 2013;100(3):608–14.
15. Schoolcraft WB, Katz-Jaffe MG. Comprehensive chromosome screening of trophectoderm with vitrification facilitates elective single-embryo transfer for infertile women with advanced maternal age. *Fertil Steril.* 2013;100(3):615–9.
16. Palini S et al. Genomic DNA in human blastocoele fluid. *Reprod Biomed Online.* 2013;26(6):603–10.
17. Gianaroli L et al. Blastocentesis: A source of DNA for preimplantation genetic testing. Results from a pilot study. *Fertil Steril.* 2014;102(6):1692–9.
18. Tobler KJ et al. Blastocoel fluid from differentiated blastocysts harbors embryonic genomic material capable of a whole-genome deoxyribonucleic acid amplification and comprehensive chromosome microarray analysis. *Fertil Steril.* 2015;104(2):418–25.
19. Magli MC et al. Preimplantation genetic testing: Polar bodies, blastomeres, trophectoderm cells, or blastocoelic fluid? *Fertil Steril.* 2016;105(3):676–83.
20. Capalbo A et al. Diagnostic efficacy of blastocoel fluid and spent media as sources of DNA for preimplantation genetic testing in standard clinical conditions. *Fertil Steril.* 2018;110(5):870–9.

21. Neal SA et al. High relative deoxyribonucleic acid content of trophectoderm biopsy adversely affects pregnancy outcomes. *Fertil Steril.* 2017;107(3):731–6.
22. Hammond ER, Shelling AN, Cree LM. Nuclear and mitochondrial DNA in blastocoele fluid and embryo culture medium: Evidence and potential clinical use. *Hum Reprod.* 2016;31(8):1653–61.
23. Kuliev A, Zlatopolsky Z, Kirillova I, Spivakova J, Cieslak Janzen J. Meiosis errors in over 20,000 oocytes studied in the practice of preimplantation aneuploidy testing. *Reprod Biomed Online.* 2011;22(1):2–8.
24. Mastenbroek S, Twisk M, van der Veen F, Repping S. Preimplantation genetic screening: A systematic review and meta-analysis of RCTs. *Hum Reprod Update.* 2011;17(4):454–66. Erratum in: *Hum Reprod Update.* 2013; 19(2):206.
25. Rubio C et al. Preimplantation genetic screening using fluorescence in situ hybridization in patients with repetitive implantation failure and advanced maternal age: Two randomized trials. *Fertil Steril.* 2013;99(5):1400–7.
26. Rubio C et al. In vitro fertilization with preimplantation genetic diagnosis for aneuploidies in advanced maternal age: A randomized, controlled study. *Fertil Steril.* 2017;107(5):1122–9.
27. Vaiarelli A et al. Biochemical pregnancy loss after frozen embryo transfer seems independent of embryo developmental stage and chromosomal status. *Reprod Biomed Online.* 2018;37(3):349–57.
28. Garcia-Herrero S et al. Embryo aneuploidy screening with CGH arrays in the absence of implantation. *Méd de la Rep.* 2014;16(2):112–9.
29. Bianco K, Caughey AB, Shaffer BL, Davis R, Norton ME. History of miscarriage and increased incidence of fetal aneuploidy in subsequent pregnancy. *Obstet Gynecol.* 2006;107(5):1098–102.
30. Pellicer A et al. In vitro fertilization plus preimplantation genetic diagnosis in patients with recurrent miscarriage: An analysis of chromosome abnormalities in human preimplantation embryos. *Fertil Steril.* 1999;71(6):1033–9.
31. Rubio C et al. Incidence of sperm chromosomal abnormalities in a risk population: Relationship with sperm quality and ICSI outcome. *Hum Reprod.* 2001;16(10):2084–92.
32. Mateu E et al. High incidence of chromosomal abnormalities in large-headed and multiple-tailed spermatozoa. *J Androl.* 2006;27(1):6–10.
33. Mateu E et al. Aneuploidies in embryos and spermatozoa from patients with Y chromosome microdeletions. *Fertil Steril.* 2010;94(7):2874–7.
34. Rodrigo L et al. Testicular sperm from patients with obstructive and nonobstructive azoospermia: Aneuploidy risk and reproductive prognosis using testicular sperm from fertile donors as control samples. *Fertil Steril.* 2011;95(3):1005–12.
35. Rodrigo L et al. Impact of different patterns of sperm chromosomal abnormalities on the chromosomal constitution of preimplantation embryos. *Fertil Steril.* 2010;94(4):1380–6.
36. Munné S, Sandalinas M, Magli C, Gianaroli L, Cohen J, Warburton D. Increased rate of aneuploid embryos in young women with previous aneuploid conceptions. *Prenat Diagn.* 2004;24(8):638–43.
37. De Souza E, Halliday J, Chan A, Bower C, Morris JK. Recurrence risks for trisomies 13, 18, and 21. *Am J Med Genet A.* 2009;149A(12):2716–22.
38. Yang Z et al. Selection of single blastocysts for fresh transfer via standard morphology assessment alone and with array CGH for good prognosis IVF patients: Results from a randomized pilot study. *Mol Cytogenet.* 2012;5(1):24.
39. Scott RT Jr et al. Blastocyst biopsy with comprehensive chromosome screening and fresh embryo transfer significantly increases in vitro fertilization implantation and delivery rates: A randomized controlled trial. *Fertil Steril.* 2013;100:697–703.
40. Forman EJ, Li X, Ferry KM, Scott K, Treff NR, Scott RT Jr. Oocyte vitrification does not increase the risk of embryonic aneuploidy or diminish the implantation potential of blastocysts created after intracytoplasmic sperm injection: A novel, paired randomized controlled trial using DNA fingerprinting. *Fertil Steril.* 2012;98(3):644–9.
41. Jobanputra V, Sobrino A, Kinney A, Kline J, Warburton D. Multiplex interphase FISH as a screen for common aneuploidies in spontaneous abortions. *Hum Reprod.* 2002;17(5):1166–70.
42. Treff NR, Tao X, Ferry KM, Su J, Taylor D, Scott RT Jr. Development and validation of an accurate quantitative real-time polymerase chain reaction-based assay for human blastocyst comprehensive chromosomal aneuploidy screening. *Fertil Steril.* 2012;97(4):819–24.
43. Treff NR, Levy B, Su J, Northrop LE, Tao X, Scott RT Jr. SNP microarray-based 24 chromosome aneuploidy screening is significantly more consistent than FISH. *Mol Hum Reprod.* 2010;16(8):583–9.

44. Yan L et al. Live births after simultaneous avoidance of monogenic diseases and chromosome abnormality by next-generation sequencing with linkage analyses. *Proc Natl Acad Sci U S A*. 2015;112(52):15964–9.
45. Fiorentino F et al. Development and validation of a next-generation sequencing-based protocol for 24-chromosome aneuploidy screening of embryos. *Fertil Steril*. 2014;101(5):1375–82.
46. Zheng H, Jin H, Liu L, Liu J, Wang WH. Application of next-generation sequencing for 24-chromosome aneuploidy screening of human preimplantation embryos. *Mol Cytogenet*. 2015;8:38.
47. Kung A, Munné S, Bankowski B, Coates A, Wells D. Validation of next-generation sequencing for comprehensive chromosome screening of embryos. *Reprod Biomed Online*. 2015;31(6):760–9.
48. Huang J, Yan L, Lu S, Zhao N, Xie XS, Qiao J. Validation of a next-generation sequencing-based protocol for 24-chromosome aneuploidy screening of blastocysts. *Fertil Steril*. 2016;105(6):1532–6.
49. Friedenthal J et al. Next generation sequencing for preimplantation genetic screening improves pregnancy outcomes compared with array comparative genomic hybridization in single thawed euploid embryo transfer. *Fertil Steril*. 2018;109(4):627–32.
50. Shamonki MI, Jin H, Haimowitz Z, Liu L. Proof of concept: preimplantation genetic screening without embryo biopsy through analysis of cell-free DNA in spent embryo culture media. *Fertil Steril*. 2016;106(6):1312–8.
51. Xu J et al. Noninvasive chromosome screening of human embryos by genome sequencing of embryo culture medium for in vitro fertilization. *Proc Natl Acad Sci U S A*. 2016;113(42):11907–12.
52. Feichtinger M et al. Non-invasive preimplantation genetic screening using array comparative genomic hybridization on spent culture media: A proof-of-concept pilot study. *Reprod Biomed Online*. 2017;34(6):583–9.
53. Vera-Rodriguez M et al. Origin and composition of cell-free DNA in spent medium from human embryo culture during preimplantation development. *Human Reprod*. 2018;33(4):745–56.
54. Ho JR et al. Pushing the limits of detection: Investigation of cell-free DNA for aneuploidy screening in embryos. *Fertil Steril*. 2018;110(3):467–75.
55. Rubio C et al. Origin of false positives and false negatives in non-invasive preimplantation genetic testing for aneuploidies. *Fertil Steril*. 2018;110(4):e412.
56. Hammond ER et al. Characterizing nuclear and mitochondrial DNA in spent embryo culture media: Genetic contamination identified. *Fertil Steril*. 2017;107(1):220–8.
57. Lane M et al. Ability to detect aneuploidy from cell free DNA collected from media is dependent on the stage of development of the embryo. *Fert Steril*. 2017;108(3):e61.
58. Kuznyetsov V et al. Evaluation of a novel non-invasive preimplantation genetic screening aproach. *PLoS One*. 2018;13(5):e0197262.
59. Li P et al. Preimplantation genetic screening with spent culture medium/blastocoel fluid for in vitro fertilization. *Sci Rep*. 2018;8(1):9275.
60. Hardy K, Spanos S, Becker D, Iannellli P, Winston RML, Stark J. From cell death to embryo arrest: Mathematical models of human preimplantation embryo development. *Proc Natl Acad Sci U S A*. 2001;98(4):1655–60.
61. Magli MC, Albanese C, Crippa A, Tabanelli C, Ferraretti AP, Gianaroli L. Deoxyribonucleic acid detection in blastocoelic fluid: A new predictor of embryo ploidy and viable pregnancy. *Fert Steril*. 2019;111(1):77–85.
62. Bolton H et al. Mouse model of chromosome mosaicism reveals lineage-specific depletion of aneuploid cells and normal developmental potential. *Nat Commun*. 2016;7:11165.
63. Van Opstal D et al. Origin and clinical relevance of chromosomal aberrations other that the common trisomies detected by genome-wide IPS: Results of the TRIDENT study. *Genet Med*. 2018;20(5):480–5.
64. Pertile MD et al. Rare autosomal trisomies, revealed by maternal plasma DNA sequencing, suggest increased risk of feto-placental disease. *Sci Transl Med*. 2017;9(405).

11

Preimplantation Genetic Testing in the Future

Joe Leigh Simpson, Svetlana Rechitsky, and Anver Kuliev

CONTENTS

Introduction

Preimplantation genetic testing (PGT) has already passed what has been labeled Version 1.0 (fluorescence *in situ* hybridization [FISH], polar body, and cleavage-stage biopsy era). Our current version 2.0 constitutes 24-chromosome testing, next-generation sequencing (NGS), and trophectoderm biopsy. Yet this too will change. Our current practice will not remain static. What, then, can we expect going forward?

Verification of Results by Cell-Free DNA in Maternal Plasma

At present we "test" embryos. We do not "screen." Embryos subjected to PGT are either transferred or discarded. Follow-up confirmation is not performed routinely, for which reason the term preimplantation genetic screening (PGS) was not considered as the correct designation [1,2]. Thus, current nomenclature consists of PGT, PGT-aneuploidy (PGT-A), PGT-monogenic (PGT-M), and PGT-structural (PGT-SR) [1,2].

It would indeed be desirable to confirm that PGT results accurately characterize the embryo. We believe this will be the first of our future predictions to become clinical practice. Methodology already exists—cell-free DNA in maternal plasma. The principle is based on DNA transcripts existing in maternal plasma, derived from both mother and fetus. Analysis of cell-free DNA to detect fetal aneuploidy is currently performed on an estimated 2 million of the 4 million pregnancies in the United States annually, an estimated 4 million of the 18 million Chinese, and in an estimated 10 million pregnancies globally.

Distinguishing a fetal trisomic pregnancy from a euploid pregnancy is based on total number of transcripts of a specific number (13, 18, 21) in maternal plasma. This total quantity is compared to that of a normal DNA reference standard. It is not necessary to separate maternal from embryonic transcripts. One simply counts the total number of transcripts for all chromosomes. Then, one compares this for each individual chromosome—13, 18, 21, in particular. A small but quantifiable excess compared to reference DNA will exist if the fetus is trisomic. Analysis of cell-free DNA detects trisomies 21, 13, and 18 at high rates for trisomies 21 and 18, 99.9% and 98% respectively [3–5].

In processing maternal plasma samples to detect DNA for liveborn trisomies, DNA information for other autosomes is unavoidably obtained. These results are at present not reported routinely, i.e., filtered. If "unfiltered," PGT-A results on all chromosomes would be known and used to confirm PGT-A results. Analytical validation is underway to generate cell-free DNA platforms suitable for reporting results of all 24 chromosomes. This methodology could be used to confirm PGT-A results in ongoing pregnancies.

Confounding factors in using cell-free DNA to confirm PGT-A include false positive results due to demise of a co-twin, maternal neoplasia, or systemic maternal diseases. False negative results can occur when the fraction of fetal DNA is less than 4%. Normal results with chorionic villus sampling (CVS) or amniocentesis can provide reassurance in these cases, but chorionic villi and amniotic fluid cells are also indirect measures of fetal/embryonic status. Neither method assesses DNA that will differentiate into fetal organs.

In conclusion, noninvasive cell-free DNA analysis based on maternal plasma will soon be available to confirm PGT-M results in ongoing pregnancies.

Cell-Free DNA to Determine if a Miscarriage was Aneuploid or Euploid

Approximately 5% of pregnancies undergo miscarriage after PGT-A. The assumption has usually been that the miscarriage was euploid and due to non-chromosomal etiology. Thus, there is no diagnostic error, yet this is not actually known. Knowing chromosomal status would allow verification that the PGT-A lab result was indeed correct, and the pregnancy lost for other reasons. This approach would be best applicable to single-embryo transfer and a singleton pregnancy.

A corollary relates to chromosomal status of products of conception. Here the impediment has long been that a karyotype requires successful cell culture. Thus, the preferred methodology at present is chromosomal microarray (CMA), which does not require cultured cells. However, either karyotype or CMA requires collecting abortus maternal, an unpleasant and not always successful task. Infection is a problem in culturing tissue, and inadvertent inclusion of maternal tissue can be an impediment with either CMA or karyotype. All this has resulted in low compliance, informative results approximating only 50%–60%.

If 24-chromosome Noninvasive Prenatal Screening (NIPS) becomes widespread, PGT-A results can be routinely verified using cell-free DNA analysis for all chromosomes in a pregnancy ending in miscarriage following PGT-A. This should actually be easier to assess in miscarriages than in ongoing pregnancies because the fetal fraction will almost certainly be sufficient [6]. In clinical miscarriages, embryonic demise occurs 2–3 weeks before clinical manifestations of pregnancy loss (so-called "missed abortion"). During this interval, placental tissue is undergoing autolysis. The fetal DNA fragments released into the maternal circulation result in a higher proportion of fetal DNA than in ongoing pregnancies. Thus, detection of aneuploidy should be easier.

In conclusion, assessing cell-free DNA on the basis of quantitative DNA increases or decreases in maternal plasma will be routine. This will enable a euploid loss to be distinguished readily from an aneuploid loss.

Selecting Embryos to Transfer through Cell-Free DNA in Culture Media

Maternal plasma can be used to accurately assess embryonic status of either ongoing pregnancies or miscarriages. Might not one use the same approach to select transferrable embryos by noninvasive methods? Promising reports exist, correlating results from analysis of culture media with results from a trophectoderm biopsy [7,8].

Major problems include achieving a sufficient embryonic fraction of DNA. This caveat mirrors the need for cell-free DNA in ongoing pregnancies to achieve 4% fetal fraction. The converse problem is that media may be "contaminated" with maternal DNA from maternal cumulus cells, resulting in the need for proportionally more fetal DNA. In addition, human serum is added to some commercially available culture media.

In conclusion, a truly noninvasive approach—embryonic DNA in media—that would bypass embryo biopsy is attractive. However, we remain wary that this approach can supplant trophectoderm biopsy and direct embryonic assessment.

Automation for Safer Embryo Biopsy

In any surgical procedure, prowess varies from individual to individual. The first "case" is rarely completely optimal. Surgeons are well aware that a learning curve must be traversed before competence is achieved. This trajectory is evident to anyone who has ever performed surgery or ever performed a laboratory procedure like embryo biopsy. Unfortunately, not all individuals who perform a biopsy are equally skilled or become so at the same velocity.

Many currently automated laboratory procedures (e.g., pipetting) were once performed by hand, using technicians having varying levels of expertise. Today, automation performs equivalent work with highly consistent results; 96-well platforms do not require 96 manual pipettings. Automated embryo biopsy will be developed and provide portability, lower cost, and replication. In fact, the entire sequence from biopsy to result could be automated.

A related question is the embryonic stage at which biopsy will occur. Will trophectoderm biopsy remain the stage of choice? Certainly this seems preferable to cleavage-stage biopsy, but obtaining DNA from or closer to the inner cell mass would be even better, if safe.

In conclusion, trophectoderm biopsy will remain the most utilized but will be obtained by automated biopsy.

PGT-M to Interrogate Genes Essential for Organogenesis

With culture media, ovulation stimulation, and embryo transfer becoming optimized, one might expect livebirth rates in ART to be 80%–90%, yet no registry reports such rates. A likely explanation is our scientific "unknown unknown"—lack of knowledge concerning the single (protein coding) genes responsible for cell lineage and differentiation. Just as congenital anomalies in liveborns may be due to perturbation of many single genes or polygenic factors, these same etiologies can be assumed to play roles in lack of success in PGT-M or PGT-A. A well-known example of an embryonic gene is OCT 4, required beyond the four-cell embryo. It can be expected that many genes pivotal for cell lineage and differentiation will become known, and will be interrogated into PGT-M or cell-free DNA platforms to select embryos that will increase liveborn results in ART. This would be analogous to targeted organ system platforms (e.g., skeletal), whole-exome sequencing (WES), or whole-genome sequencing (WGS) in chorionic villi or amniotic fluid cells.

Although many mammalian genes of potential relevance could easily be hypothesized, obtaining data directly on human embryos remains daunting. For only one-third of the 21,000 protein-coding genes is function known. We can confidently assume many of the two-thirds play roles in embryogenesis and if perturbed would explain euploid miscarriages. Once known, it would be possible to test using PGT-M. Evidence exists, in fact, that euploid miscarriages show some of the same aberrant features expected of aneuploid embryo [9,10]. Using array CGH and embryoscopy on a cohort of early miscarriages [9,10], Feichtinger et al. [10] reported that most first trimester euploid miscarriages are characterized by growth retardation or developmental abnormalities. Only one quarter appeared morphologically normal. As DNA or RNA sequencing costs continue to plummet, we can expect WES and WGS results on miscarriage cohorts. Agnostic testing will reveal genes that can be aggregated into panels and interrogated to identify those not recommended for transfer.

In conclusion, it is possible now and increasingly will be to detect single-gene euploid perturbations explaining lack of embryo development. Embryos not recommended for transfer can be identified by PGT-M. The result will be "take home baby" rates of perhaps 80%.

Expanded Carrier Screening Leading to PGT-M for Disorders of Childhood Onset

Over 600 different disorders have been subjected to PGT-M, but many more are potential candidates. At least 1000 autosomal recessive conditions could be indications for PGT-M. In the United States, monogenic disorders account for an estimated 10% of pediatric hospitalizations and 20% of childhood deaths.

Initially, PGT-M for monogenic disorders was performed because a couple had an affected child (proband). The very first PGT cases were for this indication, either X-linked (ornithine transcarbamylase [OTC] deficiency) or autosomal recessive (cystic fibrosis) conditions. In such disorders, a parent or parents could be deduced to be obligate heterozygotes, at 25% risk for another affected child. Thus, subsequent testing pregnancies was indicated.

The alternative to waiting for birth of an affected index case has long been carrier screening in the asymptomatic general population. Screening initially was ethnicity-based, undertaken for Sickle cell anemia in Africans and African Americans, B-thalassemia for Mediterranean populations (e.g., Italians, Greeks) and Tay-Sachs disease for Ashkenazi Jewish populations. Ethnicity-based carrier screening initially utilized gene products to detect heterozygosity, e.g. ratio of the enzymes hexosaminidase A and B in Tay-Sachs disease.

At present, carrier screening is no longer an exclusively ethnicity-based approach but has become pan-ethnic and DNA based [11,12]. "Expanded" screening may involve partners of different ethnicities, identifying many more at-risk couples. Information is DNA-based and thus can be sought on hundreds of genes. Determining carrier status is based on searching for causative alleles, for targeted sequencing of exons known already to contain a pathogenic variant, and for copy number variants (CNV) [11,12]. In 2018 Counsyl (2016 *JAMA* and 2018 *Clin Chemistry*) reported results of their expanded (Foresight™) panel, which at that time included 254 genes. One in 22 couples were at risk for a fetus with a detectable disorder; 1 in 300 fetuses were affected.

Expanded carrier screening has concomitantly led to an increase in PGT-M. In 2016, 38% of PGT-M cases at Reproductive Genetic Innovations LLC in Northbrook, IL were ascertained by carrier screening; the majority were undertaken following an affected proband. In 2018, 63% of PGT-M cases at RGI were ascertained by carrier screening.

In conclusion, expanded carrier screening has resulted in increased numbers of PGT-M for childhood monogenic disorders. The demand will continue to increase, especially in countries in which screening is largely independent of national health services or regulatory restraints. PGT centers worldwide offering PGT-M can expect a commensurate increase in PGT-M cases.

Increased PGT-M for Adult-Onset Disorders

In addition to pan-ethnic panels for genetic disorders of childhood onset, other panels target adults at risk for heritable adult-onset disorders. Foremost are those that screen/detect heritable cancers. Many heritable cancers are autosomal dominant, and interest is not infrequently kindled by a family member having been detected as having such a cancer. At-risk relatives often wish to be tested, and if having the mutation, avoid transmitting the mutant allele to their own offspring.

PGT-M for adult-onset cancer at RGI was performed in 65 cycles in 2016, increasing to 118 in 2018. The cancer most commonly undergoing testing was BRCA1/2, occurring in 271 of 792 cycles for PGT-M cancer. Other frequently encountered cancers include familial adenomatous polyposis 1, Fanconi anemia, neurofibromatosis, tuberous sclerosis, and hereditary nonpolyposis colon cancer (HNPCC). Adult-onset PGT-M is also increasingly undertaken for cardiac disorders (long Q-T syndrome, hypertrophic cardiomyopathy, dilated cardiomyopathy) and for neurodegenerative conditions (early-onset Alzheimer, Huntington disease).

In conclusion, screening for heritable adult-onset disorders is increasingly applied in families who wish to undergo PGT-M to identify unaffected embryos for transfer. These carriers wish their offspring not to inherit a mutant allele, using PGT-M. An increase in PGT-M cycles for adult-onset disorders is a safe prediction.

PGT and Gene Editing

Gene editing (GE) is a sentinel advance in science, genetics, and reproduction. The preimplantation embryo is well-suited for application. There is also clear rationale for GE in certain circumstances. In some cycles there are no transferable embryos, but affected embryos may exist. Affected embryos are at present discarded. If GE were available and efficacious, a "corrected embryo" could instead be transferred to achieve a pregnancy. A debate at the 2018 International Society for Prenatal Diagnosis (ISPD) meeting explored this topic [13]. Salutary reasons for GE were enumerated by Wells; Vermeesch provided contrary arguments that included low efficacy and potential off target effects. A concern distinct from safety and efficacy was that germline correction is almost unavoidable.

On the other hand, recounting history reminds us that objections have been raised to virtually every advance in prenatal genetic diagnosis. Rarely do these concerns persist. Amniocentesis was deemed dangerous in the 1960s despite being widely practiced by obstetricians of that pre-ultrasound era. Objections were raised to the concept of PGT-A and PGT-M. Especially contentious was the pioneering work of Verlinksy, Rechitsky, and colleagues to identify and transfer HLA-matched embryos for umbilical cord–derived stem-cell transplantation [14]. This indication is now well accepted in the United States, Turkey, and elsewhere. Objection to PGT-M for adult-onset disorders (e.g., heritable cancers) also exists in certain venues, but as noted is already increasing in the United States.

Prenatal genetic diagnosis and new indications for PGT thus often evoke disquiet. Once initiated, however, acceptance is almost always gained. We believe this will occur as well for GE. Initially we were optimistic that GE would not befall the hackneyed calls for a moratorium to generate "more studies." (This almost never seems to result in new data or epiphanies of wisdom.) The U.S. National Academies (Sciences; Medicine) expressed reservations over GE in 2017 but advocated research under suitable oversight [15]. The Nuffield Council on Bioethics in 2018 likewise encouraged ongoing research [16]. Both of these authoritative bodies espoused the need for safety, efficacy, and public discourse. Unfortunately, GE recently conducted in China evoked worldwide concerns over premature application, arguable indications, and incomplete oversight [17]. Although we still lack details on what was actually performed and whether truly successful, dissent must be acknowledged. This will delay clinical application. Yet the major concerns about GE—low efficiency, off-target deleterious effects—are already being addressed with evident amelioration, albeit not perfection [18]. Attraction for applying GE to cancer and other conditions remains and will eventually overcome calls to restrict access.

In conclusion, GE is not at present ready for "prime time," but neither will its benefit be denied. We cannot predict time of clinical application, but we can be confident that GE will be a component of PGT in the future.

REFERENCES

1. Zegers-Hochschild F et al. The International Glossary on Infertility and Fertility Care. *Hum Reprod.* 2017;32(9):1786–801 (simultaneous publication).
2. Zegers-Hochschild F et al. The International Glossary on Infertility and Fertility Care. *Fertil Steril.* 2017;108(3):393–406 (simultaneous publication).
3. Norton ME et al. Cell-free DNA analysis for noninvasive examination of trisomy. *N Engl J Med.* 2015;372(17):1589–97.
4. Bianchi DW, Platt LK, Goldberg JD, Abuhamad AZ, Sehnert AJ, Rava RP; MatErnal bLood IS Source to Accurately diagnose fetal aneuploidy (MELISSA) Study Group. Genome-wide fetal aneuploidy detection by maternal plasma DNA sequencing. *Obstet Gynecol.* 2012;119:1–12.
5. Zimmermann B, Hill M, Gemelos G. Noninvasive prenatal aneuploidy testing at chromosomes 13, 18, 21, X and Y, using targeted sequencing of polymorphic loci. *Prenat Diag.* 2012;32:1233–41.
6. Lim JH et al. Cell-free fetal DNA and cell-free total DNA levels in spontaneous abortion with fetal chromosomal aneuploidy. *PLOS ONE.* 2013;8(2):e56787.
7. Xu J et al. Noninvasive chromosome screening of human embryos by genome sequencing of embryo culture medium for *in vitro* fertilization. *Proc Natl Acad Sci U S A.* 2016;113:11907–12.

8. Feichtinger M et al. Non-invasive preimplantation genetic screening using array comparative genomic hybridization on spent culture media: A proof-of-concept pilot study. *Reprod Biomed Online.* 2017;34:583–9.

9. Philipp T, Kalousek DK. Generalized abnormal embryonic development in missed abortion: Embryoscopic and cytogenetic findings. *Am J Med Genet.* 2002;111(1):43–7.

10. Feichtinger M, Wallner E, Hartmann B, Reiner A, Philipp T. Transcervical embryoscopic and cytogenic findings reveal distinctive differences in primary and secondary recurrent pregnancy loss. *Fertil Steril.* 2017;107:144–9.

11. Haque IS, Lazarin GA, Kang HP, Evans EA, Goldberg JD, Wapner RJ. Modeled fetal risk of genetic diseases identified by expanded carrier screening. *JAMA.* 2016;316(7):734–42.

12. Hogan GJ et al. Validation of an expanded carrier screen that optimizes sensitivity via full-exon sequencing and panel-wide copy number variant identification. *Clin Chem.* 2018;64(7):1063–73.

13. Wells D, Vermeesch JR, Simpson JL. Current controversies in prenatal diagnosis 3: Gene editing should replace embryo selection following PGD. *Prenat Diag.* 2019;39(5):344–50.

14. Verlinksy Y, Rechitsky S, Schoolcraft W, Strom C, Kuliev A. Preimplantation diagnosis for Fanconi anemia combined with HLA matching. *JAMA.* 2001;285:3130–3.

15. National Academies of Sciences, Engineering, and Medicine; National Academy of Medicine; National Academy of Sciences; Committee on Human Gene Editing: Scientific, Medical, and Ethical Considerations. *Human Genome Editing: Science, Ethics, and Governance.* (US): National Academies Press; 14 Feb 2017.

16. Nuffield Council on Bioethics. *Genome Editing and Human Reproduction: Social and Ethical Issues.* July 2018. http://nuffieldbioethics.org/project/genome-editing-human-reproduction

17. Rana P. How a Chinese scientist broke the rules to create the first gene-edited babies. *WSJ.* May 10, 2019.

18. Eguizabal C, Montserrat N, Izpisua Belmonte JC. Repairing the damaged embryo: CRISPR-Cas9 technology. *Fertil Steril.* 2018;110(2):230–4.

Index

A

ABGC, *see* American Board of Genetic Counseling
Accreditation Council for Genetic Counseling
    (ACGC), 12
aCGH, *see* Array comparative genomic hybridization
ACMG, *see* American College of Medical Genetics and
    Genomics
ACOG, *see* American College of Obstetricians and
    Gynecologists
Acrocentric chromosomes, translocations with, 64
ADO, *see* Allele dropout
Adult-onset disorders, PGT-M for, 154
Advanced maternal age (AMA), 26, 34, 141
Agilent Technologies, 59, 85, 91
Allele drop-in (ADI), 90
Allele dropout (ADO), 29, 30, 79, 80, 88, 90
AMA, *see* Advanced maternal age
American Board of Genetic Counseling (ABGC), 12, 22
American College of Medical Genetics and Genomics
    (ACMG), 20
American College of Obstetricians and Gynecologists
    (ACOG), 20
American Society of Reproductive Medicine (ASRM),
    14, 20
Amniocentesis, 16, 18, 38, 62, 123, 155
AmplideX FMR1 PCR Kit® (Asuragen), 3
Anaphase lagging, 35, 113, 127
Aneuploid-aneuploid mosaic embryos, 112
Aneuploid embryos, 5, 6, 58, 100, 102, 120, 139
    in blastocoelic fluid, 38
    euploid and, 103
    morphokinetics of, 68, 103
    temporal delay in, 101
Aneuploid sperm, 67
Aneuploidy, 14, 34, 100, 139
    detection, time-lapse for, 39–40
    forms of, 34
    impact on embryo development, 101–102
    meiotic, 129
    in preimplantation embryos, 34
    rates, 16, 61, 66
    risk classification model, 103
    screening techniques, 14, 142
    segmental, 35, 37
    transfer of blastocysts with mosaic, 17
Angelman/Prader-Willi syndromes, 90
Annexin 5 (ANXA5-M2 haplotype), 4
Apoptosis, 146, 147
Array comparative genomic hybridization (aCGH), 15, 26,
    32, 50, 52, 70, 114, 129, 134, 142
    for classifying embryos, 131
    next-generation sequencing, 62–63

in PGT-SR, 59–60
    resolution of, 62
    SNP and, 61
Array single nucleotide polymorphism (aSNP), 114
ART, *see* Assisted reproductive technologies
ASRM, *see* American Society of Reproductive Medicine
Assisted reproductive technologies (ART), 98
    genetic counselors in, 13, 20–21
    incorporating genetic counseling services in, 21
    PGT-A and time-lapse monitoring in, 106–107
Automation, for embryo biopsy, 153
Autosomal chromosomes, 122
Autosomal recessive (cystic fibrosis) conditions, 154

B

Bacterial artificial chromosomes (BAC), 32, 59–60
BAF, *see* B-allele frequency
Balanced carriers, 62, 68, 70
Balanced rearrangements, 50
    complex chromosomal rearrangements, 56
    insertional translocations, 56
    inversions, 54–56
    reciprocal translocations, 50–54
    Robertsonian translocations, 54
    types of, 50–56
B-allele frequency (BAF), 84, 90
BasePhasing, 61, 62, 69–70
BF, *see* Blastocele fluid
Biopsies
    blastocentesis, 140
    blastocyst biopsy, 140
    blastomere biopsy, 140
    PB biopsy, 140
    timing, 27
    types of, 140–141
Biopsy mosaicism, 17
Blastocele fluid (BF), 38
Blastocentesis, 38–39, 140
Blastocoel fluid, 57, 140
Blastocyst, 29, 37, 101
    biopsy, 101, 140
    mosaicism, 133
Blastocyst-stage (trophectoderm) biopsy, 28–29
Blastocyst-stage embryos, 34, 61, 63, 67, 119
Blastocyst-stage mosaicism, 36
Blastocyst-stage multicellular biopsies, mosaicism
    detection in, 117–118
Blastomere
    biopsy, 15, 28, 63, 83, 102, 140
    from cleavage-stage embryos, 27
BlueFuse Multi software (Illumina), 32, 59–60
Bureau of Labor Statistics, 12

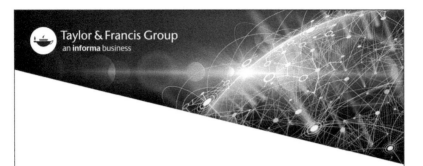